Edgar Cayce's

Guide to Colon Care

Edgar Cayce's
Guide to Colon Care

Sandra Duggan RN

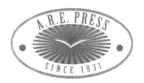

A.R.E. Press • Virginia Beach • Virginia

The contents of this publication are intended for educational and informative use only. They are not to be considered directive nor as a guide to self-diagnosis or self-treatment. Before embarking on any therapeutic regimen, it is absolutely essential that you consult with and obtain the approval of your personal physician or health care provider.

Cover design by Christine Fulcher

DEDICATED
To
SAI BABA

Contents

Acknowledgments

With special thanks and deep appreciation to:

BARBARA

JAN

KAREN JANINE DAVIS
for her inspiration, friendship, and pre-chapter quotations

DORIS VAN AUKEN
for her patience, encouragement, and editorial assistance

Preface

For forty-three years, Edgar Cayce (1877–1945) provided clairvoyant, medical diagnoses and treatment suggestions for thousands of people who requested readings. His psychic source drew on a vast knowledge of herbs, nutrition, hydrotherapies (colonics, steam/fume baths, whirlpool baths, etc.), osteopathy, mechanical and electrical devices, and much more. Usually twice a day, he would lie down on a couch, go into a trance state, contact the unconscious mind of an individual and Universal Consciousness, and respond to the seeker's questions. The response was then transcribed by Cayce's secretary.

These readings are available to the public. Names have been replaced with numbers to preserve the privacy of the individuals who received the readings. For example, if a person's first reading is numbered (2056-1), the second reading will be (2056-2), and so on. Of the 14,256 readings given, almost 9,000 are on the topic of health.

The A.R.E., the Association for Research and Enlightenment, is a non-profit membership organization formed in 1931 to preserve and research the readings. The A.R.E. Library/Conference Center houses the largest collection of documented psychic information in the world. The A.R.E. offers such member benefits as a newsletter, a magazine titled *Venture Inward*, lessons for home study, and a lending library by mail. Study groups meet in private homes worldwide and apply the Cayce material for personal growth. Conferences and seminars are offered year round, and the Visitor Center has daily tours; free lectures on dreams, meditation, healing, and other topics; a movie on Cayce's life; and audiovisuals and exhibits. The bookstore and the Cayce/Reilly® School of Massage are also open to the public.

The readings on colonics are indexed in the A.R.E. library under "Intestines: colonics," in the card catalog. About 1350 readings were given on colonic irrigation, 500 on colon problems, 1000 on enemas, 10 on diarrhea, 300 on colitis, 175 on constipation and almost 2900 on laxatives. Cayce obviously had a great deal to say about the importance of colon health.

For twenty years, colonics, massage, and other hydrotherapies were available at the A.R.E. Therapy Department, which opened in 1966. As you may know, it was directed by Dr. Harold J. Reilly, D.Ph.T., D.S., a physiotherapist (one who uses physical and mechanical remedies, such as massage, hydrotherapy, electricity, heat, etc. in the treatment of disease) who also held degrees in naturopathy and chiropractic, and completed two years of osteopathy. He studied with John Harvey Kellogg, M.D., of Battle Creek, Michigan, and owned the Reilly Health Institute in Rockefeller Center, New York City.

In January of 1920, a woman came to see Reilly, saying that she had been specifically referred by Cayce, in a reading, to have massage and hydrotherapy with Dr. Reilly. Reilly had never heard of Edgar Cayce, and could not understand how Cayce knew not only his name, but also the therapies he offered in his practice. The two finally met in person two years later and developed a close, working partnership. Reilly himself had several readings from Cayce, and learned that he had spent many past lives as a healer, working with massage and hydrotherapy. Reilly continued to work with the guidance given in the readings long after Cayce's death, for he fully believed in drugless therapies that allow the body to heal itself. Reilly was a good example of health and productivity and lived well into his nineties.

Dr. Reilly "retired" from his practice in 1966, became Director of the A.R.E. Therapy Department and donated all of his equipment: Dierker colonic machines, massage tables, a whirlpool bath, and two porcelain Sitz baths.

In 1986, the Therapy Department closed and the Cayce/Reilly School of Massotherapy was founded. It offers both a 225-hour and a 600-hour program teaching the Cayce-Reilly method of massage, hydrotherapy, Cayce remedies, sports massage, anatomy/physiology, and related body therapies. In May of 1995, the Therapy Department was reborn as the Health Services Department of the A.R.E., offering massage, hydrotherapy (including colonics), and related services.

ONE

My Involvement

The body of each entity is the temple of the living God. There He has promised to meet the entity. To live, to be—and that activity—unto the glory of the Creative Forces is the purpose of the entrance of each entity into material consciousness.

2981-1

My involvement with colon health and colon irrigation began the day I was interviewed for the position of Supervisor of the A.R.E. Therapy Department. Along with 250 other members who were also nurses, I had received a letter saying there was a position available. It just so happened that I was going to be passing through Virginia Beach and could conveniently stop by.

I had only recently learned about Edgar Cayce and, just prior to this, had been reading everything I could find on Egypt, dreams, and spiritual subjects. But my knowledge of holistic health was still in its infancy. When I learned that my prospective job was to administer colonic irrigations and supervise the massage therapists, I had no idea what was required. Not wanting to risk losing the opportunity for employment, it seemed wiser to ask, "What's a colonic?" before things got more complicated. This was to become a very familiar question over the years, for many people have very little knowledge about colon health and colonics. Though this form of hydrotherapy is recognized as a highly beneficial approach to alternative health care not only by Edgar Cayce, but also by such varied holistic health care professionals as osteopaths, naturopaths, chiropractors, acupuncturists, massage therapists, and many others, the medical profession seems to be either unaware or misinformed about colon irrigation. At any rate, a colonic sounded simple enough—it was some sort of internal bath that used a professionally designed machine to give a high irrigation of the colon, or large intestine. My background as a nurse was helpful, but not really necessary for certification as a colon therapist.

My first day at the A.R.E. was a memorable experience. It was not difficult to run the colonic machine, but actually giving a colonic was much more involved, for no two colons nor colonics are alike. My first client, who had never had a colonic before, was even more nervous than I was! We both lived through it, however, and he felt so much better he made another appointment. In contrast, my next client had been getting colonics as a health maintenance therapy for twenty years, and tried to teach me all about colon health as she directed her colonic, step by step. She also shared her struggles in trying to keep her colon healthy, which was an ongoing problem for her.

Suddenly, there was an urgent request for an appointment from an A.R.E. conferee. She had not had an elimination in four days, and was not feeling well. I was to learn that this is a fairly common problem when someone is traveling or on vacation. The combination of sitting all day, not drinking enough water, and not stimulating the lymph through exercise changes the patterned condition of eliminations.

And so the day went. I learned more about the importance of a happy, healthy colon in one day than I had in my whole lifetime.

Bursitis

Working at the A.R.E. was life-changing for me, as well. Apparently, I was not there just to help others. Within a month, I developed acute bursitis in my right shoulder, and it became hot, swollen, and painful. The accompanying discomfort in the muscles of my arm made the problem even worse. From a medical standpoint, bursitis generally results from a build-up of calcium deposits, and becomes painful when the shoulder is overused. The tendency is then not to move the arm, which can result in a stiff or frozen shoulder.

Bursitis tends to happen when we feel very stressed and overburdened with responsibilities we have "shouldered." At that time, I was unaware that emotions had anything to do with the physical health of the body, and simply thought that I had moved the handle on the colonic machine too much.

A friend suggested that I apply castor oil packs (these will be explained in detail in Chapter 8) without heat, since the area was already hot and inflamed. This did bring a measure of comfort and relaxation to my shoulder muscles, but the problem remained. Someone in the department informed me that a local chiropractor always prescribed colonics for her bursitis patients—a series of two colonics a week for a three-week period because she recognized that bursitis is caused by colon problems as well as a poor diet. I had never had any colon problems, and at that point knew very little about diet, other than that it was something you went on occasionally to lose weight. Besides, what did the colon have to do with a shoulder problem? They weren't even in close proximity to each other.

So, not understanding how the colon affects everything in the body, I decided to go for a cortisone injection that would *really* work. Much to my surprise, it only took away the sharp edge of the pain, leaving a dull ache. However, what helped the most was that the doctor actually massaged the muscles in my arm and shoulder for five minutes. It was the first time I had ever experienced any form of massage, and it made me realize how much of my discomfort had been caused by tense muscles. Nevertheless, the bursa was still painful and my shoulder could not be moved.

Two days later, our receptionist took it upon herself to schedule me for six colonics. I gave up and agreed. Now it was *my* turn to be on the receiving end, literally, and learn what colon cleansing was all about. There was no noticeable difference until the fourth colonic, when I experienced a subtle movement in the colon on the right side near the hepatic flexure. A few moments later, it seemed as if something also moved in the most painful area of my shoulder. Amazingly, I was able to raise my arm about 120° without any difficulty. The pain and discomfort had been considerably alleviated, and the whole area felt different. During the fifth colonic, there was another movement in the same area of the colon, and all of the residual pain left my shoulder. Afterwards, I was able to move it around in a full range of motion, and I felt as if my shoulder were "back." Needless to say, I decided to make a commitment to routinely follow up with maintenance colonics at the change of seasons, and to discover, as well, what food patterns had contributed to the problem. Although there have been intermittent periods of stress in my life, I have never again experienced bursitis.

I later researched the readings on bursitis, which clearly attribute the disturbance to a build-up of matter in the pockets of the colon, blocking reflexes to the shoulder and causing pressure. This explained why a series of colonics was necessary to help loosen the build-up, and why it felt as if something had actually moved in the colon. Indeed, in the course of my colonic, when the water finally loosened old fecal matter, energy was unblocked and my shoulder was freed.

Reflex Points

The concept of reflexology, which states that there are reflex points in the feet, hands, and ears that correspond to various organs, glands, and areas in the body, is fairly well known. However, it is not generally understood that there are reflex points in the colon, as well.

If you could grasp the colon by the cecum and hold it straight up, these points would line up in direct correspondence with the head and trunk of the body.

Reflexology has been influenced by acupuncture and oriental healing therapy, which holds that the body/mind is created, maintained, and works by energy. This "Ki," (also known as *chi*) meaning *life force* or *energy flow*, circulates throughout the body along invisible meridians. There are points on these meridians where the energy gathers and is particularly active. The large intestine meridian, for example, which has 20 points, runs from the index finger of each hand up both arms to the nose.

Colon Reflex Points

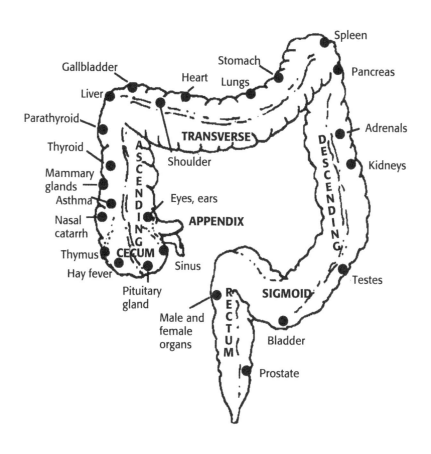

**Adapted from Colon Health
by Norman Walker, D.Sc., p. 10.**

Colon Held Straight Up

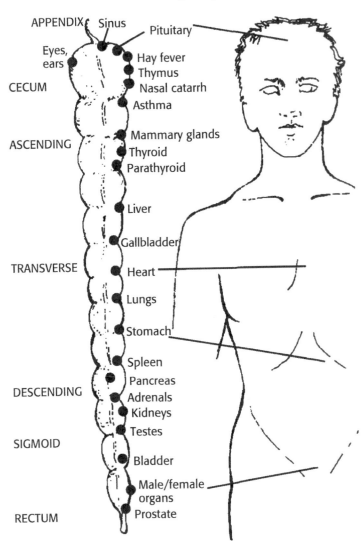

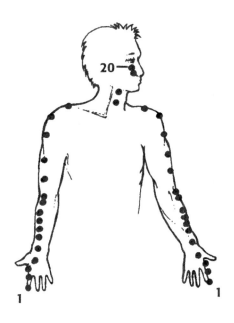

When the Ki becomes unbalanced or blocked from injury, stress, or illness, this ultimately creates a disharmony in the internal glands and organs. To restore balance, needles are inserted into the specific meridian points to release energy, relieve discomfort and pain, and maintain health.

Other oriental therapies, such as acupressure and Shiatsu, are less invasive and stimulate the points with thumbs, fingers, elbows, and knees. Foot and hand reflexology use specific hand and finger techniques to alternately press points and rebalance the energy flow. It is this same effect that is accomplished in the colon as the colonic water removes matter and mucus, and gently stimulates points to release energy.

Back Pain

One day a middle-aged man hobbled into the reception room. He was bent over from back pain, could hardly walk, and had been scheduled for surgery the next day. The prescription narcotic he was taking was very constipating, and at his wife's insistence, he had come to us for a colonic. The man was miserable, and grumbled about everything and everyone, including his wife, who had gotten him into this "unbelievable situation." Near the end of the colonic, he let out a whoop and exclaimed that his back pain was gone! I couldn't believe it and neither could he! He waltzed out, kissed his wife, and cancelled the surgery. Since he had a history of sluggish eliminations, he decided, on his own initiative, mind you, to schedule a series of colonics and begin to work on his colon health.

Not all back pain is caused by a full colon, nor relieved so quickly, but it can happen. Eric Mein, M.D., in *Keys to Health: The Promise and Challenge of Holism*, explains that if the colon is engorged or distressed by being constipated or overfull, it may irritate the nerves of the lumbar area of the back and cause muscle spasms. By removing the solid matter in the colon, pressure on nerves is released, muscles relax, and pain is relieved.

The opposite effect, however, can also occur. If there is an injury to the lumbar area, any swelling, inflammation, or muscle spasms will put pressure on spinal nerves that affect the colon. The result is poor eliminations. In this case, cleansing the colon will relieve the constipation, but will not alleviate the back pain as dramatically.

Over the years, many people have been helped by following the advice given in the readings to have colonic irrigations. It almost seems too simplistic, but then Cayce's drugless therapies *are* simple. What is difficult is motivating ourselves to follow the advice. I know, for many of my clients, it was initially like climbing a mountain just to muster the courage to call for an appointment. Fear of the unknown is a great stumbling block. But many also asked afterwards, "Is that all it was?"

People have shared with me their stories of how colon cleansing has changed their lives. Some related that by cleansing their colon, they could now accept that it was time to begin their path of healing. Truly, I have received my *real* education from all the wonderful people who have undertaken a path of self-transformation, and for that, I remain eternally grateful.

Summary

1) A colonic is an alternative health hydrotherapy that gradually and gently cleanses the colon pockets and stimulates muscle tone.

2) Bursitis is caused by negative emotions, poor diet, and poor elimi-nations. The build-up of matter and mucus in the colon blocks re-flexes to the shoulder and causes pressures there.

3) There are reflex points in the hands, feet, ears, and colon that affect internal organs and glands. Reflexology has been influenced by acu-puncture, which holds that Ki or life force energy runs along invisible meridian lines in the body.

4) Ki energy becomes blocked from injury or stress and can be re-stored by inserting acupuncture needles into appropriate points along the meridians.

5) Acupressure, Shiatsu, and hand and foot reflexology stimulate the points with thumbs and fingers to release energy blocks.

6) Irrigating the colon may relieve symptoms when lower back pain is aggravated by a distended colon.

TWO

Colon Health

Remember, the whole body—physically, mentally, spiritually— is one; and it is as each portion of the system coordinates with the other that there is the better attaining of the normal balance and activity.   *920-13*

There is only that necessary, for the full physical normal condition, to keep the mind and body active, and to keep the eliminations near normal. This is, as we find, necessary in every physical being.   *265-33*

One of Edgar Cayce's greatest contributions to health education is his teaching that basic health begins with colon health, and that a poorly functioning colon can cause disease.

As I worked with the colon, I came to realize that our society has a serious lack of colon health. More Americans today are hospitalized with problems and diseases of the intestinal tract than any other area of the body. Most of these problems were unheard of 100 years ago, for in earlier times, people's diets consisted of stoneground whole grains and high-fiber foods. Around 1880, however, the amount of fiber, bran and wheat germ used in flour production decreased because of "improved" milling methods. Today, we are left with a flour product that contributes very little to nutritional needs.

At the same time that flour was being processed more, people left the farms and moved to the cities where food now had to be shipped in. There was a new demand to preserve food for longer periods. Over the years, various technologies—from canning, freezing, and dehydration to today's methods of refrigeration and irradiation—were developed to prevent food spoilage and increase shelf life. These methods of processing food reduce enzymes, vitamins, and the life force of food. Although food keeps longer this way, it cannot support optimal life. All of this contributes further to the decline in colon health. The tragedy is that most colon disease can be prevented with a diet of whole grains, fruits and vegetables, and non-processed foods.

Lung and colon cancer are two of the most common forms of cancer in this country. This pairing is not surprising to the oriental mind, for it is well known in their culture that the lung and large intestine meridian are very closely connected. One of my clients, when in his early thirties, found this to be especially relevant. He had been experiencing pressure in his chest accompanied by shortness of breath. Since nothing could be found medically to cause his symptoms, he decided to try an alternative holistic approach. Dietary changes (omitting caffeine sodas, fried food, and white flour products) and an exercise program of working out with weights to expand his lung capacity all helped. But when he discovered colonics, and settled into a program of colon cleansing twice a year, there were no further problems.

Taboo Subject

Many people are not inclined to discuss the subject of eliminations. We are often taught that bowel movements are dirty and, as a result, we learn to ignore or reject the whole process. Many who really need help with colon problems are often the most reluctant to seek it. Perhaps they were forced to have enemas as a child to relieve constipation or help ward off a cold, for there was a time when enemas were routinely given at the first sign of illness. Before antibiotics, for example, when a patient was admitted to the hospital, the first thing a doctor ordered was a high enema. Often, this was sufficient to reduce toxicity, bring down a fever, and completely change the course of an illness. I have also come to learn that cleansing the colon helps to heal negative feelings and old emotional traumas, for water is SPIRIT and brings LIGHT into the *soul*, as well as into the dark areas of the colon.

Normal Stool

Fecal matter, or stool, is composed of about 75% water; the rest is solid, indigestible material. A normal stool is soft, firm, breaks up easily, is light or medium brown, and floats on the water. If it sinks, it is loaded with mucus, and is thought to be a constipated stool even if there is a daily elimination. Since mucus is sticky and slimy, it packs the stool more tightly and lengthens the time it takes to pass through the colon. Consequently, more pushing and straining may be necessary to have an elimination. A healthy stool is quickly eliminated and fully formed. It should not be hard and round, or thin, like a pencil.

The color of the stool, which is produced by bile pigments in the liver, is often affected by the food that is eaten or some medicines, such as Pepto-Bismol. Beets, for example, have been the culprit behind many a panic-stricken phone call to me, proclaiming, "I passed some blood in my stool!" Beets have a way of turning the urine pink for a day or two, as well.

Normal Eliminations

There is a great deal of confusion and disagreement when it comes to defining a normal elimination. Some colon books say that there should be an elimination through the alimentary canal three times a day. This may happen if someone is on a raw food diet, but such is generally not the case. On the other hand, many doctors feel that a person's bowel pattern is normal even if eliminations occur only three or four times a month. Edgar Cayce saw things differently. He said that there should be at least one good, thorough elimination each day. As one gets older and has less physical activity, it becomes even more important to have a full, daily elimination. He did not explain what "thorough" or "full" meant, but it is generally understood that the sig-

moid and descending colon, that together are about 1½ to 2 feet long
and 2 to 2½ inches in diameter, should empty with each bowel movement.

There is also a great deal of confusion and misunderstanding about
the location and shape of the stomach, small intestine, and colon. For
example, people often rub their abdomen below the navel, and mis-
takenly complain that they have a stomachache, when what they really mean is that they have gas pains in their intestines or colon, or are
feeling constipated. The stomach itself is on the left side of the body
underneath the lower ribcage. Some people have some very odd no-
tions about the shape of these organs, as well. An elderly man initially
asked why I was massaging the right side of his "stomach" during his
colonic. When I explained that I was massaging his colon, which is
shaped like an upside down "U," he related that he had always thought
it was shaped like a balloon.

Intestinal Bacteria

The colon contains 400–500 varieties of bacteria, fungi, yeast, and
viruses. The normal balance should be about 80–85% "friendly"
lactobacteria (L. acidophilus, L. bifidus, bulgaris, brevis, and saliveria)
and 15–20% putrefactive bacteria (E. coli, B. welchii, and B. putreficus,
for example), which emit toxins and gas. The friendly bacteria produce
vitamins and digestive enzymes that help control the E. coli and keep
it in balance. With the typical American diet and use of antibiotics—
which kill the intestinal bacteria as well as the infection—the balance
can be reversed to as much as 85% E. coli and only 15% lactobacteria!

Friendly bacteria thrive in such fermented foods as apple cider vinegar, miso (soybean paste), sour pickles, sauerkraut, kefir, sourdough
products, and healthstore yogurt. (The yogurt available in health food
stores is generally of a higher quality than that found in local grocery
stores, and does not contain sugar.) If there is a problem with systemic
yeast or Candida, care should be taken to avoid these foods until there
is no longer an overgrowth of yeast. (See Chapter 12 for more information.)

Although acidophilus comes in a liquid or capsule form, the cheap-
est and most vital source is Rejuvelac. This fermented, whole grain

product can be made at home using the freshest supply of whole wheat berries or millet. The wheat berries will last ten days, but the millet must be discarded and replaced every four days. The liquid Rejuvelac tastes sweet, like whey, and should not be used if it smells or tastes bad.

HOW TO MAKE REJUVELAC

Thoroughly scrub a measuring cup with hot, soapy water and rinse thoroughly just before using.

Add 2½ cups purified or distilled water to 1 cup whole wheat berries or millet. Cover and leave at room temperature for 1½ days.

Strain off the liquid (this is the Rejuvelac) and refrigerate. Drink ½ cup with meals and discard any extra liquid.

Immediately add 1½ cups more water to the grain, cover, and leave at room temperature for 24 hours.

Each day for 10 days, pour off the liquid, refrigerate, and add another 1½ cups water to the grain.

Transit Time

The length of time it takes for food to be ingested, processed by the stomach and small intestine, and eliminated by the colon is called the transit time. This process normally takes 14–18 hours when the colon is healthy and the bowel contents move along quickly. However, many people who only eliminate every three to four days have a transit time of 72–96 hours. This slow passage of stool allows toxins to be reabsorbed, pathogenic bacteria to build up, and parasites to thrive in decaying, stagnant matter.

A simple way to determine transit time is to first eat something that can be clearly identified in the stool. For example, the ingestion of charcoal capsules or tablets (these can be purchased from a pharmacy or health food store) will show up as black in the stool; beets, of course, give a reddish color. Be sure to note the time when the identifying substance (capsule or food) is taken and when the discoloration appears in the stool.

Water

Drinking enough water each day—pure water, stressed Cayce—is vital to colon health. Finding a source of pure water is even more of a challenge today. If there is not an adequate intake of water, the stool dries out, causing constipation and toxic overload of the capillary blood circulation. Cayce often stated that sufficient water intake—generally six to eight glasses a day—(not soda, fruit juice, coffee, or tea) would help correct constipation.

How and when water is consumed is just as important as the quantity. Liquids should be taken up to thirty minutes before a meal or two hours afterwards, so the digestive enzymes will not be diluted. Instead of chewing our food thoroughly, we have a tendency to wash it down with liquids. Cayce said this habit of bolting food causes more colds than any other poor diet practice.

To aid digestion, alkalinize the system, help the eliminations, and prevent poisons from accumulating in the system, the readings often suggest squeezing the juice from a rolled lemon (pressing while rolling the lemon back and forth on a hard surface to loosen the juice inside) into a glass of body–temperature water and drinking it at least 30 minutes before breakfast.

Diet

The colon can be cleansed, but if there is not a shift in eating patterns afterwards, then problems can recur. Diet is discussed in depth in Chapter 5, for it is one of the most important factors in colon health. As adults, we are solely responsible for what we eat, and we make choices every day that impact our lives. Sometimes we consciously choose not to make changes, even if it means shortening our life. Such was the case for a 69–year–old woman (1840) who requested a reading on March 8, 1939. She was experiencing indigestion, heart problems, shortness of breath, and weakness. Cayce found that a plethoric condition (excessive blood in the walls) of the ascending colon was the cause of poor circulation between the heart, liver, and lungs. The treatment was simple:

Gradual colonic irrigations every three days. (The third irrigation would relieve the pressure on her heart and lungs.)

No potatoes or macaroni and cheese. No red meat; only chicken and fish.

Vegetables eaten raw at times, and cooked in Patapar Paper at other times.

Sadly, in a follow-up report, a friend said that the woman had died a year after the reading, and never followed the guidance because she felt she could not live without potatoes.

Exercise

A daily program of brisk walking in the morning when the dew is on the ground is the best kind of exercise, according to Cayce, for "it is using the energies that enable the body to produce better eliminations of toxic forces" (3155-2). Apparently, there is a higher vibrational energy at that time of day. The oxygen and ozone in the fresh, outdoor air keep the blood flow balanced through the lungs, heart, liver, and kidneys.

The colon is also much happier with some form of regular exercise, such as walking or bicycling. Biking helps massage the colon as the thighs alternately press on the ascending and descending colon.

Cayce generally recommended that vertical exercises and deep breathing be done first thing in the morning to bring more oxygen into the lungs in preparation for the activities of the day. (During sleep, the breath normally becomes very light and shallow.) A vertical exercise is any circular or stretching movement of the head, neck, shoulders, elbows, wrists, hands, or waist when standing or sitting.

Horizontal mat exercises were advised to help normalize circulation and take the strain off of blood vessels in the legs after working all day. Dr. Harold J. Reilly, in *The Edgar Cayce Handbook for Health through Drugless Therapy*, says that the following horizontal exercises will help reduce the abdomen and stimulate the organs in that area. "They also help to tighten the muscles, to control the forming of pockets or diverticulitis in the large colon, and to correct constipation" (p. 132, large paperback edition).

He recommends beginning any exercise program by doing each exercise six times, then increasing by two each week until totaling twelve. It is vitally important to coordinate the breath with each movement.

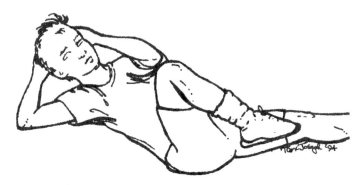

Elbow-Knee Kiss
- Lie on your back and clasp hands behind head.
- Inhale.
- Exhale as you bend the right knee and the upper body to touch left elbow to the right knee.
- Hold 3–6 seconds.
- Inhale as you release and return to starting position.
- Repeat with opposite knee and elbow.

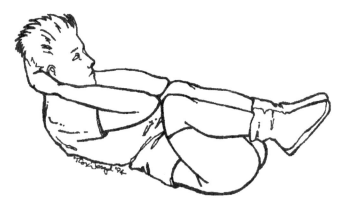

Double-Knee Kiss
- Lie on your back and clasp hands behind head.
- Inhale
- Bring both knees up to both elbows as you exhale.
- Hold for 3–6 seconds.
- Inhale as you slowly return to starting position.
- Do four times, then add one time each week until you reach 12.

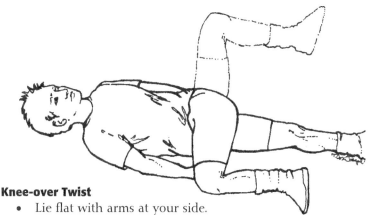

Knee-over Twist

- Lie flat with arms at your side.
- Bring left knee up to a 90° angle as you inhale.
- Keeping shoulders flat, twist at the waist and bring leg over to right side as you exhale.
- Hold for 3 seconds.
- Inhale as you bring leg back up.
- Exhale as you slowly return to starting position.
- Repeat with other leg.

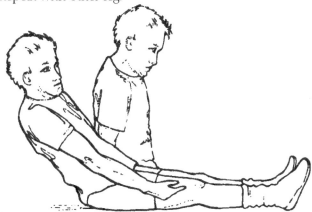

Sitback

THIS IS POTENTIALLY DANGEROUS TO WEAK BACKS. DO WITH SUPERVISION.

- In a sitting position, inhale and hold head down with chin on chest.
- With legs stretched out in front of body, and arms at sides, exhale as you lean back to a 45° angle while keeping chin on chest. Hold for 3–6 seconds.

- Inhale as you come back up.

This is a particularly good exercise for women to tighten the muscles of the lower abdomen. It keeps pressure off the lower pelvic girdle, increases circulation, gives movement to the organs, glands, and intestines, and pulls sagging organs up into their proper position.

Summary

1) Basic health begins with colon health, for a colon that is not functioning properly causes dis-ease and eventually disease.

2) Enemas used to be routinely given for illness in children and hospital patients to reduce fever and change the course of an illness.

3) Cleansing the dark areas of the colon helps heal old emotional traumas and brings in Spirit and Light.

4) Edgar Cayce suggested that there should be at least one good, thorough elimination each day.

5) A normal stool is light to dark brown, about 1½ to 2 feet long, floats on water, and is fully formed.

6) Preparing one's own Rejuvelac is an economical way to obtain vital, live lactobacilli.

7) Cayce suggested drinking six to eight glasses of pure water each day.

8) It is necessary to support colon cleansing with appropriate dietary changes.

9) Take brisk, daily walks in the early morning when the dew is on the ground.

10) Deep breathing and vertical exercises should be done in the morning and horizontal exercises done in the evening.

11) Dr. Reilly recommended several horizontal exercises to strengthen the abdomen, control diverticulitis, and correct constipation.

THREE

Anatomy and Physiology

For as indicated ever, there is gradually a replenishing of every portion of the body, if the proper balance is kept in the system so that the eliminations and assimilations are such that each portion of the system may reproduce itself.   *4061-1*

The intestinal tract consists of the esophagus; stomach; small intestine, which is approximately 20–22 feet in length and 11½ inches in diameter; and the large intestine or colon, which is 4–5 feet long and 2½ inches in diameter.

Purpose of the Intestines

The small intestine originates at the pyloric end of the stomach and connects to the colon 20–22 feet later at the ileocecal valve. (See the diagram on page 24.) Its purpose is to digest and absorb food.

The first section, known as the duodenum, is where pancreatic digestive enzymes and bile mix with food. Peristaltic movements slowly move the chyme, or liquified food, along. Nutrients are absorbed into the bloodstream through five million finger–like projections and folds

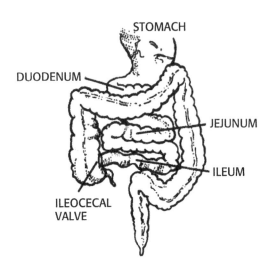

called *villi*, which line the walls. Cayce often speaks of the lacteals, the villi that absorb fats. The lacteals connect with the lymphatic system and empty into the return circulation to the heart.

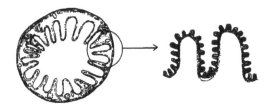

The second section of the small intestine is the jejunum (6–12 feet long; 8 foot average), and the last section is the ileum (9–18 feet; 12 foot average). Nodules of lymph tissue called *Peyer's patches* are found here, which contain lymphocytes whose purpose is to attack any bacteria that manage to survive coming into contact with the hydrochloric acid in the stomach. As we grow older, the hydrocholoric acid diminishes, and the villi and Peyer's patches begin to atrophy, impairing the process of assimilation. So even though the diet may be in balance, the nutrients are not being absorbed properly. A series of castor oil packs (see Chapter 8) applied three to four times a year can help to maintain the health of the small and large intestine by stimulating the flow of lymph in these areas.

As chyme reaches the end of the ileum, it must then pass through a valve into the cecum (the first section of the colon). This ileocecal valve is normally closed, but opens as chyme reaches it. Any water from an enema or colonic does not go back through this valve into the small intestine if the valve is functioning properly.

The purpose of the colon, or large intestine, is to absorb electrolytes and excess water from the chyme and form a solid waste product. The friendly colon bacteria are able to manufacture vitamin K and some B vitamins, such as B_{12}, riboflavin, and thiamine, in a healthy colon.

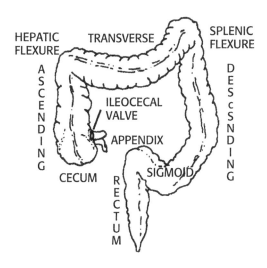

Sections of the Colon

CECUM

The cecum is a 2½-inch blind pouch that forms the first part of the colon. The appendix, a 3- to 6-inch long, finger-like pouch, extends from the cecum.

ASCENDING COLON

This section is wider near the cecum and narrows as it approaches a

90° bend called the *hepatic (liver) flexure.* Chyme must move slowly uphill against gravity, and then make a sharp turn. If eliminations are sluggish, the ascending colon can become very distended and congested.

TRANSVERSE COLON

This is the largest and most movable section of the colon. It makes another 90° bend on the person's left side, called the *splenic (spleen) flexure.* It will sag or prolapse from the weight of solid matter remaining in the colon too long.

DESCENDING COLON

The colon then descends 5 to 6 inches before connecting to the sigmoid section.

SIGMOID

This is the narrowest part of the colon and is approximately 16 inches long. It is shaped like an "S" to prevent solid waste matter from emptying too quickly into the rectum.

RECTUM

This final part of the colon is approximately 12 inches long. It has an opening called the anus, which has two sphincters to help control the evacuation of stool.

Pockets

A smooth, mucous membrane lines the villi–free walls of the colon. A small amount of alkaline mucus is secreted from glands in the wall,
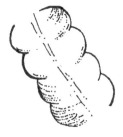
protecting the delicate lining from too much acidity or abrasive waste matter. The colon has many pouches or pockets, called *haustras,* which contain layers of muscle that allow the colon to expand whenever necessary to accommodate varying amounts of solid matter. These muscles regularly make rhythmic contractions and re-laxations called *peristalsis,* that slowly mix and move the bowel contents along.

Summary

1) The purpose of the colon is to absorb water from the liquid, digested food (chyme) and form a solid waste product. If the colon is healthy, bacteria will manufacture vitamin K and some B vitamins.

2) Villi line the walls of the small intestine and assimilate nutrients from the digested food.

3) The colon has no villi. It contains glands that secrete a small amount of mucus to protect the delicate membranes from too much acid and abrasive material.

4) The colon has smooth–shaped pockets called *haustras* that expand or contract during peristalsis to move the bowel contents along.

FOUR

Why Cleanse?

If a cell is left in the system that should be eliminated, or if it IS of that condition of inactivity, then all the cells gathered about it cannot heal that cell. It must produce sufficient of the lymph or leukocyte, that condition which will gather about it and move it out of the system, to let the new supply take its place!

Hence we have that called coagulation, or incoordination, producing distresses from a bad coordinating elimination in this body.   243-7

Why should we cleanse this five-foot-long colon that goes uphill against gravity, makes a sharp turn, frequently sags in the middle, makes another sharp turn, and then goes downwards? After all, isn't it supposed to clean itself whenever there is an elimination? Not so, said Cayce, who emphasized that the colon should periodically be irrigated with water.

For *every* one—everybody—should take an internal bath occasionally, as well as an external one. They would all be better off if they would.   440-2

Many of the physical problems that develop over the years can *easily* be avoided by a high–fiber diet and occasional colonics to clean out the accumulation of matter in the colon pockets and keep the colon muscles toned.

Case History

In 1938, a 51–year–old spinster school teacher requested a health reading (1703-1). She asked about diet, her reliance on coffee, and wanted help with an exercise program. She was worried that she was too thin and lacked vitality. She particularly wanted to know if she had cancer, tuberculosis, a tumor, or any dead material in her body that would account for her excretions having such a bad odor.

Now, here was a woman who was advanced spiritually and quite knowledgeable about health matters. Her long letters to Cayce give exact details about her symptoms and reactions to the advice given in the readings. To improve her health, she had spent thousands of dollars on cleansing diets and fasts, electrical health machines, massage, osteopathy and naturopathy treatments, and health spa fees. She exercised daily, took nude sun baths, and drank raw juices. However, the one area where her health was sadly lacking was the colon. She had been constipated since childhood, and relied on laxatives and enemas, although they were no longer "doing the job."

She told Cayce that she had recently gone to a "painless, bloodless surgeon" who found that her abdominal organs sagged, and that the colon was "tied down" with adhesions. (These commonly occur after abdominal surgery, when the peritoneal lining becomes glued together and constricts the intestines and colon.) The surgeon was very concerned, and felt there was a tendency for cancer to develop because the colon was in such poor condition. No wonder there was a foul odor to her stool! In order to cure her, he recommended abdominal surgery to lift the sagging organs and remove the adhesions.

Rather than spend $510 for surgery, which would be equivalent to thousands of dollars today, she asked Cayce for help. He found no evidence of tuberculosis, but said there were indeed cancer cells in her body. Instead of forming a tumor, they had apparently been "kept distributed" all over her body by her various attempts over the years to fast and cleanse. She was walking a very fine line, however, for her vital forces were in a state of deterioration.

A longstanding condition of mucus in her head, throat, and digestive system prevented food from being assimilated, which, in turn, kept her weight at roughly 90 pounds. The extreme toxicity from years of constipation not only interfered with her vision, but created a condition of hyperacidity that periodically caused canker sores.

Cayce recommended the Wet Cell appliance (a low-voltage, high-vibrational battery) and steam/fume baths with pine oil, followed by a Swedish massage. A special oil formula was to be massaged into the nervous system (cerebrospinal and autonomic) along both sides of the spine, from the first cervical to the sacrum. At the end of the treatment, an alcohol rubdown was to be given to the whole body.

Codiron, a combination of cod liver oil and iron, was recommended, as well as dietary advice that was *"most necessary"* warned Cayce, for some of the health diets she had followed had been too hard on her system. She was overjoyed to learn that *if* she followed all the suggestions, her abdominal organs would be lifted, and the adhesions would dissolve without the need for surgery.

Her letters give a fascinating account of her trials and tribulations in attempting to follow the suggestions given in her reading. She argued with Cayce when his advice didn't agree with her own ideas of what she considered right for herself. For example, she wanted to remain a vegetarian for spiritual reasons, and could not bring herself to eat fish, fowl or lamb, nor to drink beef juice. She preferred distilled water and fresh raw juices to Cayce's non-carbonated Coca-Cola syrup that was recommended to help prevent the formation of gas. She also resisted using the Wet Cell appliance, and could not understand why he would not sanction the use of her own electrical machines. This seems to be a case of someone who really wanted help, but was simply unable to accept any advice contrary to her own.

A check reading, or follow-up reading, given two months later, noted that she refused to follow some suggestions, and urged that everything be carried out persistently and consistently in order for healing to occur. She asked why Cayce hadn't mentioned her constipation in the first reading, and he answered that someone with her knowledge of health should have known about colon health. He then gave one of those wonderful, general statements:

> And the keeping of the colon clean is that which is necessary for
> *every* well-balanced body; hence should be and is a part of the
> experience for each entity.   1703-2

This concept that a clean colon is vital to our health and well–being
is an extremely important and crucial one. If the body can be kept free
of toxic build–up, then it is capable of normally assimilating nutrients,
and can replenish itself. Cayce went even further to say that, with a
proper balance in the assimilations and eliminations, there can be a
rejuvenation and longevity to whatever age we desire. As you may
recall, it was not uncommon to live to be several hundred years old
during biblical times. Each cell in the body can live indefinitely as
long as it does not become overloaded with its own waste products.
For:

> There is within the body [that] which *will* replenish if the body is
> kept cleansed from the impurities of poor eliminations. 1464-1

Colon cleansing is not a new concept, but it seems to have fallen by
the wayside in modern times. It was first recorded in 1500 B.C. in the
Ebers Papyrus, an ancient Egyptian medical document. Pliny said the
Egyptians discovered the idea of injecting water into the colon from
the example of the ibis, a sacred, stork–like bird which used its slender,
downward–curved bill for this purpose.

In *The Essene Gospel of Peace*, translated by Edmond Bordeaux Szekely,
the Hebrew sect known as the Essenes led a simple life of work, service, prayer, and meditation. They believed they were preparing for
the coming of the Messiah, and that it was necessary to have a healthy
body to aid in this preparation. An important part of their health regimen was cleansing the colon. To do so, they took a gourd with a long,
trailing stem, and filled it with warm river water. Then they kneeled
down, inserted the stem into the rectum, and called upon the Angel
of Water to help rid them of all "uncleanliness, impurities, and
abominations."

Organs of Elimination

Our body is equipped with four organs that eliminate needless waste products and toxins: the colon, kidneys, skin, and lungs. A fifth one, the liver, is the principal organ of detoxification. Since it has no external opening, it is not considered a major organ of elimination. However, it is extremely important, because everything that is taken into the stomach has to filter through the liver (except fats, which are absorbed by the lacteal system and pumped directly through the heart to the lungs—'for clarification,' as Cayce said) before entering the bloodstream. Any toxins from food, beverages, or poor digestion are then carried into the intestines by the bile manufactured in the liver and stored in the gallbladder.

All five organs must coordinate with one another for the body to eliminate properly. In Cayce's viewpoint, the colon actually does most of the work:

> The greater amount of drosses of all natures, as the common sense knows if giving it consideration, are carried through the alimentary canal. These are not the *only* sources; for the kidneys, the breath, the perspiratory system also eliminate certain drosses or poisons. But the greater amount—seventy-four percent—is usually eliminated through the alimentary canal. 257-251

If one organ becomes congested, the others have to work overtime to try to keep the system balanced. The sooner balance can be restored, the better. It is actually harmful for an organ to eliminate toxins it does not normally handle. This creates an added stress as annoying symptoms arise—a skin rash may develop, for example, or halitosis (bad breath); there may be underarm or foot odor. We have come to accept body odor as a way of life, but, ideally, it should be minimal if the body is able to adequately get rid of its wastes and toxins. Babies smell sweet and clean because of good eliminations and their simple diet of milk.

The regular use of antiperspirants blocks the underarm channels of elimination. The body then has to use other exit points, causing an overload of toxins in the colon and kidneys. Cayce's recommendation for a "deodorant" was just to wash more frequently with soap and water.

Dietary changes, fasting, steam/fume baths, and colonics all help to remove toxins and eliminate odor. A good indicator of internal cleanliness is when there is no longer any underarm odor.

Toxic Build-Up

The physical body is a machine that makes normal waste by-products of cellular metabolism, such as uric acid, lactic acid, and carbon dioxide. A healthy body easily disposes of these natural by-products. We begin to have problems when these substances, as well as toxins foreign to the body, overload the eliminating channels.

Cayce defines toxicity as follows:

> When there is the lack of eliminations of used energies, or of refuse or carbon as it might be called, or the ash of nerve and muscular forces still left in the system, it becomes toxic poison—or toxemia.
>
> Toxic poison, then, is that condition in alimentary canal, in liver, kidneys, throughout the circulation repressing the activities—owing to the quantity of ash left from body refuse not eliminated.
>
> 464-31

Some toxins have external sources, such as pesticides, food preservatives, chemicals, drugs, medicine, irradiated food, artificial sweeteners, heavy metals, and food contaminated with radio-active fallout. Other toxins are produced within the body as a result of improper food combining, overeating, poor digestion, and inadequate assimilation. We can also reabsorb our own toxins and literally poison ourselves when waste matter moves too slowly through the colon. This is called auto-intoxication. A condition of intestinal stasis and toxicity then occurs, and toxins back up into the blood and lymph.

A person's blood was generally "read" first in a physical health reading because it is such an important factor in assessing the toxicity level of the liver, colon, and kidneys. Blood purification starts in the liver. When there are too many toxins, the liver becomes overloaded and torpid (one of Cayce's favorite words, meaning *sluggish*), and is no longer able to function as an adequate filtration system. The highly-regarded Henry Bieler, M.D., author of *Food Is Your Best Medicine*, endorses this concept when he writes:

> As long as the liver function is intact, the bloodstream remains pure. When it becomes impaired, the toxins enter the circulation and cause irritation, destruction, and eventually death. (p. 68)

As his book title suggests, Dr. Bieler believes that the food we ingest determines our health—improper foods cause disease, while proper foods cure it.

The impact of toxins on the body is staggering. A 19-year-old woman (5450) asked Cayce why there were painful and disfiguring boils and abscesses on her face, legs, and skin. He found the underlying reason was poor eliminations, and that toxins had been reabsorbed into her bloodstream. This was too much for the blood to handle, so they were unloaded through the skin. A subsequent bacterial infection caused further complications. She was warned that colitis or appendicitis would develop unless radical changes were made.

The Cayce readings are full of hundreds of cases of people who sought help for all kinds of major and minor problems caused by toxins. Even a minor irritant such as sand in the eyes or scum on the teeth should be addressed immediately, for it is giving us a message that we need to do some internal cleansing, as in the following example.

A 34-year-old woman (457), who had a chronic problem of constipation and hemorrhoids, requested a reading primarily for infertility, but also because she wanted to know why there was a gray film on her teeth. Cayce informed her that her chemical balance was off because of poor eliminations, and the resulting toxins and drosses being discharged by the lungs were causing the present condition in her mouth. First and foremost, as we might expect, he suggested that the colon be cleansed. (For treatment of the mouth condition, see reading 457-11 in the Appendix.)

In another case, a 25-year-old woman (191) was suffering from tonsillitis, laryngitis, bronchitis, cough, fever, burning eyes, and a pound-

ing headache. Cayce said that all of her problems were due to poor
eliminations and drosses that had infected the liver, inactivated the
bile ducts, and produced an overabundance of blood so contaminated
that it made her sick.

The toxins also affected her nervous system, causing the "ganglia to
work in an extraordinary or an abnormal manner." The upper half of
her body was experiencing fast pulsations in the head, neck, and
palms, and the lower portion was chilly, having hot and cold sensa-
tions.

Three specific therapies were prescribed to bring about a permanent cure. (See the Appendix for reading 191-1, which also includes
the formulas specified.)

Here are some further problems caused by toxic build-up that are
mentioned in the readings:

> Stiff knees
>
> Feeling tired and listless
>
> Dizziness
>
> Headache
>
> Joint pain
>
> Muscle pain in arms and legs
>
> Poor digestion and assimilation
>
> Nerve pain
>
> Anemia
>
> Nasal catarrh (mucus)
>
> Swelling and stiffness in the hands
>
> Moodiness and irritability
>
> Allergies to fruits and vegetables
>
> A twitching in any part of the body
>
> Problems with the spinal nervous system
>
> Itchy hemorrhoids
>
> Skin rash
>
> Sluggish liver

Kidney problems

Mucus in the colon

Eye problems (iritis)

Dark circles under the eyes

Burning sensation in the eyes

Brown blotches on the face

Heart palpitations

Hypertension (high blood pressure)

Toxins can also be transferred through a mother's milk to her baby. A 22-year-old woman (136) had been getting readings for two years because of poor eliminations. Her 62nd reading was requested after the birth of her baby. She had not made much progress, for it was "still necessary that those conditions of eliminations in this body be more *thoroughly* established in their correct channels," and now her baby was being adversely affected by poisons transferred via her breast milk. She had to temporarily stop nursing, remove the toxic milk with a breast pump, and cleanse her system with laxatives.

Poor Eliminations

There is a marvelous article called "Death Begins in the Colon" by the Royal Society of Medicine of Great Britain. It states that almost every known chronic disease is directly or indirectly due to the influence of more than 30 bacterial poisons that are absorbed from the intestines. These poisons accumulate because of poor eliminations from the colon.

Dr. Bernard Jensen, D.C., author of *The Science and Practice of Iridology*, is able to clearly demonstrate this direct, reflex relationship between the toxicity of the colon and symptoms of disease or malfunction in the organs of the body through iridology, a non-invasive diagnostic tool that can determine the health or illness of the organs, glands, and other areas of the body through the study of the iris. One half of the colon is indicated in each eye: the cecum, ascending colon, and half of the transverse colon encircle the right pupil; the other half of the transverse colon, descending colon, sigmoid, and rectum encircle the left pupil.

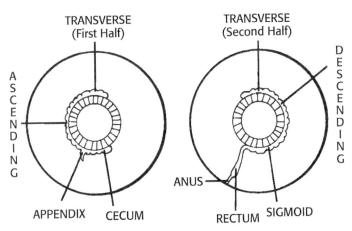

Iridology reveals where there is acute or chronic inflammation and toxic build-up in the colon wall. This manifests as enlarged, dark areas in the colon area of the iris, and each of these areas will in turn correspond with a specific organ or part of the body.

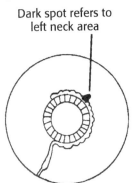

Dark spot refers to left neck area

One of Dr. Jensen's early case histories was of a woman with torticollis, or wryneck, who had been treated for five days with osteopathy, chiropractic, and physiotherapy before consulting him. She also informed him that she had been constipated for the past week, and that the left side of her colon had been sore to touch for several months. In the eye examination, Dr. Jensen found a black area in the descending colon portion of her iris, a section corresponding with the neck. Within three hours of receiving a series of enemas, almost all of her neck symptoms disappeared.

Dr. Jensen has worked with many patients in his lifetime. As a standard question in gathering medical history, he asks patients to point to the physical area in the body that troubled them *before* their illness actually manifested. In every case, they have pointed to an area in the colon. He says that abscessed teeth, lung infections, muscle problems, and cancer are *all* caused by toxic accumulations that originally come from the colon.

In his book, *Tissue Cleansing Through Bowel Management*, Dr. Jensen emphasizes that toxins must be eliminated before *any* method, no matter how sophisticated, can overcome disease in a toxin-laden body.

Mucus Build-Up

There is always a small amount of mucus present in the colon in order to help lubricate the passage of stool, but too much of an accumulation can interfere with peristaltic movement by slowing it down or even stopping it altogether. This build-up of mucus can also put pressure on reflex points. When the colon is sluggish, toxins and acidity irritate the delicate mucous membrane lining. Inflammation then occurs, causing the glands in the colon to produce more mucus as a protective measure.

Mucus comes in various shapes, sizes, and colors. It can look like confetti; large, two- to three-inch clumps that float like seaweed, or even four- to six-inch pieces of string. It can be white, yellow, beige, or even dark brown/black if it has been in the colon for a long time. With the addition of Glyco-Thymoline to the water, however, I have seen a great deal of mucus released during colonics (see Chapter 8). (Glyco-Thymoline is an alkaline antiseptic that helps to loosen and dissolve mucus.) When Cayce was asked how many colonics were necessary, he always stressed the importance of having a *series* of colonics until the mucus is eliminated. Afterwards, a maintenance program can be initiated.

Intestinal Cleansers

The walls of the colon become coated with layer upon layer of hard, dark, rubbery mucus from years of eating processed, chemicalized, mucus-forming junk food and dairy products. This lining, which interferes with the exchange of wastes from the blood into the colon, can be removed with intestinal cleansers. There are several effective products on the market that contain psyllium husks, which are preferable to the seeds. As the husks absorb water and swell, the hard mucus is dissolved and carried out of the colon as a soft, slippery mass. If there is severe constipation or a prolapsus, psyllium should not be used.

Some products also contain bentonite or volcanic ash, which lifts the hard mucus off the walls without dissolving it. Colonics, taken in conjunction with these products, help to quickly remove the old mucus so that toxins are not reabsorbed.

Other Reasons to Cleanse

Whenever there is a twinge of discomfort or disease in the muscles or organs, this is a signal that toxins are accumulating. A young woman recently came to my office for a series of colonics because she felt her colon had slowly become sluggish. After the second irrigation, she was astonished to discover that a chronic ache in her calf and Achilles tendon had magically disappeared. While reflecting on this mystery, she realized that the initial discomfort had coincided with the onset of her colon problems.

A colonic is also indicated when the spine is adjusted, for toxins are released into the lymph at this time. If the colon, blood, and lymph are already congested, these new toxins cannot be removed, and interfere with the benefit of the spinal work. Hence, it is not surprising that Cayce advised colon cleansing so that the adjustments would hold better.

It is also very important to have colonics when one is fasting or undertaking a cleansing program to rid oneself of parasites or Candida (systemic yeast). This will quickly clear the colon and prevent a healing crisis—a condition in which toxins are thrown off by the cells faster than the body can eliminate them.

And, finally, when you have been under severe stress, incurred an injury, or had surgery, remember that the level of toxicity dramatically increases. A client of mine suffered a broken nose as a result of her car being rear-ended while she was stopped at a red light. After having corrective surgery, her face was black and blue and so swollen that her eyes were almost shut. She felt and looked like she had been run over by a truck. A week later, she scheduled an appointment to "detox from the anesthesia." The immediate results of the colonic were far-reaching and absolutely incredible. By the time she was finished, her face had almost returned to its normal size and shape, and the discoloration was reduced by fifty per cent. The colonic apparently allowed the excess blood and lymph fluid to drain from her head, and she healed very quickly.

When to Cleanse

If we are fully aware and tuned in to our physical bodies, then *we* know best when to have spinal adjustments, when to fast, and when to clean the colon. Some physical warning signs indicating the need for a colonic are headaches, increased underarm odor, excessive gas, heaviness in the abdomen, or a feeling of depression. Also, any of the symptoms listed under *Toxic Build-Up* earlier in this chapter indicate that the level of toxins is building up faster than they can be effectively eliminated.

Dreams bring us messages from our subconscious mind and Higher Self to pay attention to our bodily needs when we have ignored the signs and signals on a conscious level. Usually, we have an inner knowing of their meaning for us, although there are many books available to help accurately interpret the symbology. A very common colon dream, for example, is that something is wrong with the bathroom plumbing; it is either clogged or not working properly, and the toilet can be overflowing.

A woman I know dreamed that the sewer was backing up, and water was rising in her house. She said she woke up knowing that the sewer meant her colon was blocked, and the water represented blood and lymph fluid that was filling up with toxins in her physical house.

A male client dreamed that he drove into a gas station where the word *colonic* was printed on each pump. You can't get a sign much clearer than that. If we are open and receptive, we can always get help and guidance through our intuition and dreams.

Once you have embarked upon a program of colon cleansing, you will begin to notice some significant changes. And as you begin to feel better, look younger, and have more energy, you will be inspired to maintain a healthier lifestyle.

Summary

1) Edgar Cayce said everyone would benefit by cleansing their colon occasionally.

2) You cannot expect to be healthy by fasting and following other health regimens without also having a properly functioning colon.

3) We can live as long as we desire if there is a proper balance in assimilation and elimination.

4) Colon cleansing is an ancient concept that was practiced over 2,000 years ago by the Essenes.

5) The four organs of elimination (the colon, kidneys, skin, and lungs), as well as the liver, must all coordinate together.

6) Toxic build-up from poor eliminations can cause all kinds of physical symptoms.

7) Every part of the colon has a direct relationship to specific organs of the body. This correlation is also signified in the iris of the eye.

8) Mucus build-up can clog the colon, stop peristalsis, and put pressure on points that reflex to other areas of the body.

9) Intestinal cleansers containing psyllium husks help dissolve and loosen old, hardened, rubbery mucus.

10) Our dreams often guide us when we need to pay attention to our bodily needs.

FIVE

Diet and Nutrition

Urges arise, then, not only from what one eats but from what one thinks; and from what one does about what one thinks and eats! as well as what one digests mentally and spiritually!

2533-6

Begin with the activities in the diet that will make for the resuscitating of more vital forces. Do not overfeed, so that the body becomes a dross pit—as it were; but only take sufficient that the body does assimilate, does use up *those forces that are taken into the system.*

626-1

Once a program of colon cleansing has been embarked upon, the importance of a proper diet cannot be stressed enough, for as Cayce said, "What we think and what we eat—combined together—*make* what we *are*; physically and mentally." (288-38)

The choice of what we eat is very complex, for there is no diet that is right for everyone. We learn how to eat from our parents and culture at a very young age. Food is often an emotional security blanket; we turn to food to numb our feelings, or often overeat for self-destructive reasons. As we realize how our eating patterns are making us ill, we begin to ask questions, read nutritional books, and change our lifestyle. Then, as our spiritual, mental, emotional, and physical needs change, so does our choice of food.

Cayce gave dietary advice in almost every first-time reading. He often urged people to use common sense, and to pay attention to what agrees or disagrees with the body when making a dietary change.

A thirty-five-year old man (331) wanted to know what caused his depression and how he could cure it. Cayce told him that his liver was sluggish, and a toxemia was forming in the colon. The best cure was through the diet because the system could then adjust itself. The reading went on to say that *we have the means within us to create everything to keep us vital and cure ourselves.* However, when we are unbalanced, outside forces from food or medicinal properties are needed.

The Cayce Diet

Although Cayce gave advice for specific individuals, some guidance was given so often that it can be generalized. For instance, nerve-building foods are to be eaten for breakfast and lunch, while blood-building foods are to be eaten for dinner.

BREAKFAST
- Fruit alone.
  or
- Hot or cold whole grain cereal with milk (preferably soy milk).
  or
- Coddled egg yolks with whole grain toast and butter.

LUNCH
- A raw fruit salad.
  or
- A raw vegetable salad with olive oil and lemon juice.

Although a variety of salad vegetables is mentioned in the readings, the following are to be eaten almost daily: lettuce (a blood purifier), celery, carrots, and watercress. A 23-year-old woman (480-19) was told that "the adherence to the use of carrots, lettuce, and celery EVERY day at a meal or as a portion of the meal will insure against any contagious infectious forces with which the body may come in contact."

DINNER
- Broiled or baked fish, chicken, turkey, or lamb.
- 2-3 above-ground vegetables to 1 below-ground vegetable, cooked in Patapar Paper (parchment paper—see section on vegetables, page 48).

Some Cayce Gems

ALMONDS
If two to three raw almonds with the brown skins intact are taken daily as a snack or properly combined with other food, Cayce said we need never fear cancer.

> An almond a day is much more in accord with keeping the doctor away, especially certain types of doctors, than apples. For the apple was the fall, not almond—for the almond blossomed when everything else died. Remember this is life!   3180-3

CITRUS
Citrus fruit or juice is never to be taken with cereal and milk—Cayce even said not to have them on the same day—for this combination changes the acidity in the stomach to a detrimental condition, and makes an indigestible curd. Citrus taken alone, however, acts as a laxative and is very beneficial.

EGGS
Coddled egg yolks are frequently advised in the readings. To coddle eggs, drop the yolks into a pan of boiling water, remove the pan from the stove, cover, and allow to sit for five minutes.

Unlike the yolk, egg whites are acidic, mucus-producing, difficult to digest, and act adversely on the lymph ducts in the upper alimentary canal.

CARROTS

Carrots are an exceptional food. Cayce recommended that they be eaten raw, juiced, or cooked in their own juices in Patapar Paper, almost daily. They supply vitamin B complex and many easily assimilated minerals, such as phosphorus, gold, silicon, calcium, iron, and iodine. (The presence of these minerals in the carrots, however, depends on the quality of the soil.) Carrots also purify the blood, improve the eyesight, help build the teeth, and aid the digestive forces.

In a reading for an eight-month-old baby boy (5520-2), the mother was told to rub large, cold chunks of raw carrots on the gums when the baby was teething.

GELATIN SALADS

Cayce often said that a raw vegetable gelatin salad should be eaten at least three times a week. The gelatin acts as a catalyst for the glands, and enables them to be more sensitive to vitamins. He told a 46-year-old woman (3051-6) with poor eliminations to use the top portion of the carrot, near the green stem, in her gelatin salad, for it carries vital energies that stimulate the optic reactions between the kidneys and eyes.

The Edgar Cayce Handbook for Health through Drugless Therapy, by Harold J. Reilly, offers the following recipes:

Gelatin Salad with Raw Vegetables

1 envelope unflavored gelatin
½ cup cold water
1 cup boiling water
2–3 teaspoons honey, or to taste
¼ cup lemon juice
1 tablespoon grated onion
2 cups chopped raw vegetables. Choose 3 to 4 from the following: carrots, celery, watercress, parsley, radishes, tomatoes, peas, squash, onions, chives, etc.

Dissolve the gelatin in cold water.
Add boiling water and stir thoroughly. Add honey and lemon juice,

and stir well. Add onion and vegetables, and stir well. Chill until firm.
Serve on lettuce with mayonnaise or salad dressing.

Gelatin Salad with Fruit

   1 envelope unflavored gelatin
   ½ cup boiling water
   1½ cups unsweetened pineapple juice
   1 tablespoon lemon juice
   2 tablespoons finely cut banana
   2 tablespoons chopped unsweetened pineapple
   1 tablespoon finely cut orange
   1 tablespoon finely grated coconut

Dissolve gelatin in boiling water, then boil for one minute, stirring
constantly.

Add pineapple and lemon juice and let cool. When slightly thick,
add fruit; chill until firm.

Serve on lettuce with mayonnaise or salad dressing.

Note: If one does not desire, or cannot eat, a salad, the dry gelatin can
also simply be stirred into vegetable juices and taken before it gels.

MEAT

Although Cayce was always telling people to eat more vegetables,
which "are nature's way, the natural, the correct, the cleansing," he did
not advocate vegetarianism, per se. Actually, he stressed that what
came out of a person's mouth did more harm than what went into it.

An early reading given in 1922 for a woman in her seventies (4188)
is one of the few times he did suggest that someone eat only vegetables, and it shows his rare sense of humor, as well:

Q. Mr. Cayce, should this body have any special diet?
A. Live only on those things that are green and grow above the
ground.
Q. Can this body use meat at all, Mr. Cayce?
A. That is not green. Does grow above the ground, though.

Fish, fowl, or lamb that is baked, broiled, or stewed, *never fried*, was his preferred choice of animal protein. A few individuals were told they could have well-cooked beef once or twice a month, for it has a body-building effect on the blood. However, Cayce warned against eating red or rare beef and pork, especially with acid-forming starches such as bread or potatoes, because this combination is too hard to digest.

A 45-year-old woman (443-6) wished to know if eating meat affected one's spiritual understanding. Cayce said no, not unless someone believed that it did. He went on to say that if one's ancestors had eaten meat for generations, then for them not to continue to eat some meat in this lifetime would take away from the "revivifying influences" of the body. However, he did advise others to eliminate it for their spiritual growth, especially "if that is where the spirit leads the body for the cleansing." (341-37, a 25-year-old male)

VEGETABLES
Vegetables are to be wrapped in Patapar Paper and cooked in their own juices. This is a parchment paper that does not dissolve when wet, and can be used over and over again. The vegetables are tied in a sheet of moistened paper and cooked in boiling water. They taste better when prepared in this manner, and all of the vitamins, juices, and mineral salts are retained.

When choosing vegetables for a meal, a particularly important fact to consider is how they grow. Cayce recommended a ratio of two to three above-ground vegetables to one below-ground vegetable. (Underground, tuberous vegetables contain heavy starches that are hard to eliminate.) Even then, starch content seems to be a further consideration, for Cayce also cautions against consuming too many pod vegetables, such as peas and beans, which, of course, do grow above the ground.

The following case is an exception to these general guidelines. I am including it as an example of Cayce's ability to tune in to the uniqueness of an individual's specific physical makeup and needs.

A 60-year-old male (1539) complained of low blood pressure, pain under his heart if he worked too hard, and a leg rash. Cayce found that his problems were all due to anemia that, in turn, was caused by poor assimilations *and* poor eliminations. His high level of mental anxiety didn't help matters, for it left him feeling exhausted. This lack of vitality affected his blood pressure, circulation, heart, and nervous system. One interesting suggestion made by Cayce was that he should eat *more* vegetables that grow under the ground, because the vibratory influence of the earth was needed in his healing.

Above-Ground Vegetables

Artichokes (California)	Celery	Mushrooms
	Corn	Okra
Beans	Cucumber	Peas
Broccoli	Eggplant	Peppers
Brussels sprouts	Kohlrabi	Pumpkin
Cabbage	Leafy greens	Squash
Cauliflower	Lettuce	Tomatoes

(Leafy greens include kale, collards, beet tops, parsley, mustard and turnip greens, spinach, dandelion greens, watercress, endive, Swiss chard, escarole, wild greens, etc.)

Below-Ground Vegetables

Artichokes (Jerusalem)	Radishes
	Rutabaga
Beets	Salsify
Carrots	Sweet potatoes
Celery root	Turnips
Garlic	White potatoes (eat the skin only)
Leeks	
Onions	Yams
Parsnips	

Factors That Influence Digestion

EAT REGULARLY, SLOWLY, AND SIMPLY

The habit of consistent, regular mealtimes allows a feeling of hunger to occur, which stimulates the flow of gastric juices. A 56–year–old female (243–23) was told not only to eat the right thing, but to take *time* to eat, which would allow food to digest before she again became mentally and physically active.

The stomach gets overwhelmed when too many different kinds of food are eaten together. Heartburn and indigestion are a sign that something is wrong, and antacids only mask the problem. Rather than eating a 7–grain bread or 12 ingredients from the salad bar, it would be beneficial to select a single–grain bread or 3–4 salad vegetables for one meal. This allows the digestive enzymes to work more effectively.

Following the guidelines for proper food combining (described later in this chapter) also promotes proper digestion, and alleviates the need for antacids, which neutralize the stomach acid needed to break down proteins.

NEGATIVE ENERGY

When we take in food, we also take in everything that is going on around us. If there is violence or fighting on TV or at the dinner table, that influence is absorbed along with the food. Even the habit of reading a book or newspaper during a meal has its effect; therefore, eating should be an activity in and of itself. Many spiritual communities observe silence during mealtime so that one can fully concentrate on the act of taking in food with an attitude of appreciation and prayerfulness. Food can then be eaten slowly and in harmony with the purpose for which it is being consumed.

We not only absorb the life force and vitality of the food itself, but the energy of everyone who has handled it: the seed company, the farmer, the harvester, the trucker, grocery store employees, and those who do the shopping, cooking, and serving.

Their state of mind has a tremendous impact on the food and, ultimately, on us. Therefore, we should take a few moments to quietly bless and give thanks for our food by holding our hands over it. This not only helps to uplift our conscious awareness, but also clears any negative emotions, and makes the food more compatible with the assimilation process at the cellular level. The readings also advise that a time of quiet be taken *after* meals.

Anger is especially hard on the body during digestion. Instead of being properly digested, the food produces poisons and toxins. Cayce warns us not to eat anything whenever we are angry, tired, excited, or under stress, because such states impede digestion.

COLORS OF FOOD

The colors of food not only look attractive on the plate but, more importantly, they correspond to the seven chakras or energy centers of the body and their respective colors in the rainbow. Gabriel Cousens, M.D., in *Spiritual Nutrition and the Rainbow Diet*, feels that the color of each food we eat—this means fruits, vegetables, grains, nuts and seeds, not the colors in candy or processed foods—heals, cleanses, energizes, builds, and rebalances these centers, as well as their related organs, glands, and nerve centers. Since the colon, small intestine, stomach, pancreas, liver, and spleen are all energized and affected by the second and third chakra, orange and yellow fruits and vegetables should be a major part of the diet. Although Cayce did not offer support for this theory, perhaps he didn't simply because he was never asked about its validity. I personally feel that this concept is particularly important for anyone working with colon health or any related digestion and elimination problems.

Orange Foods *(2nd Chakra, Lower Abdomen)*	*Yellow Foods* *(3rd Chakra, Solar Plexus)*
Carrots	Corn
Winter Squash	Summer Squash
Yams	Wax Beans
Sweet Potatoes	Bananas
Apricots	Pears
Peaches	Lemons
Cantaloupe	Grapefruit
Tangarines	Pineapple
Oranges	
Nectarines	
Mangoes	
Papaya	
Pumpkin	

Edgar Cayce's Chakra System

INDIGO/CROWN-PINEAL

VIOLET/PITUITARY

BLUE/THROAT

GREEN/HEART

YELLOW/SOLAR PLEXUS

ORANGE/LOWER ABDOMEN

RED/ROOT

Note: The numbering of the chakras is based on the sequence in which they are touched by energy rising from the base. The energy goes up the spine, over the top of the head, then to the brow, following the shape of the shepherd's crook or staff.

It is interesting to note that the majority of food colors are in the lower, more earthy chakras, and that there are fewer foods in the blue and lavender hues of the upper three, more spiritual centers. But have you noticed the popularity of the decorative purple kale and cabbage plant in recent years?

Diet for Proper Digestion and Assimilation

The sight, smell, and taste of food stimulate the flow of gastric juices and have a very positive influence on digestion. Digestion really starts in the mouth, so each bite should be thoroughly chewed and savored.

The readings mention salsify, rhubarb, and Jerusalem artichokes as being particularly beneficial because they create a better balance in the organs of digestion and assimilation. Salsify, also known as the oyster plant because it tastes like an oyster, is a root vegetable. It can be found wild or grown in a garden, but it is not commercially available. Rhubarb stems (also called pie plant) are a natural laxative; however, the poisonous leaves should be avoided. The Jerusalem artichoke, or sunchoke, is a tuber that looks somewhat like ginger root.

When our food is properly broken down, it can be more easily absorbed and assimilated, which allows the colon to do its job more effectively. We can further aid this process by knowing what foods combine well, and what foods are difficult to digest.

EASY TO DIGEST
- Fruits (No raw apples. No bananas if anxious or stressed.)
- Broths, simple soups
- Fish, chicken, lamb
- Milk (taken alone)
- Cereals

DIFFICULT TO DIGEST
- Fried foods
- Cheese with flour (grilled cheese sandwiches, quiche, pizza, lasagna, macaroni and cheese, cheese and crackers), cheese popcorn
- Pastries, doughnuts, cake, cookies
- White bread

- Meat, rare or red
- Soda, carbonated drinks (Cayce called them "slop for the hogs" and said they irritate the lymph.)
- Potatoes

Taking too many supplements at one time can be difficult for the body to digest and assimilate. One client of mine took ten vitamin and mineral pills with each meal. During the colonic, she saw them passing by in the observation tube of the colonic machine *in their original shape!* Much to her dismay, she realized that she had been wasting her money.

The same is true for foods that are combined improperly, such as animal protein with starch (see below). Again, this makes it difficult for the food to be broken down and assimilated, which can cause gas, belching, or heartburn.

IMPROPER FOOD COMBINING

NO animal protein combined with a starch that grows above ground (grilled cheese, hamburgers, hot dogs, quiche, pot pies, meat and bread, spaghetti and meat balls, sandwiches, cheese popcorn, chicken and rice, cereal and milk, pizza, lasagna). Combining meat and potatoes would therefore be slightly preferable to combining meat and bread, for example.

NO sweets with starch (cookies, cake, pie, doughnuts, pastries, toast with jam, pancakes with syrup, cereal with sugar).

NO coffee mixed with milk or cream (creates an indigestible curd).

NO citrus with cereal or milk (becomes acid and does not digest).

NO starch with starch. (Only one starch per meal. No pasta with bread, no bread and potatoes, etc.)

NO fried food. (Heating oil alters the fat molecules and increases the incidence of arteriosclerosis or build-up of plaque in the arteries.)

PROPER FOOD COMBINING

Animal protein with vegetables.

Bread or crackers with vegetables, nuts, seeds (hummus, peanut butter, cashew nut butter, almond nut butter, and tahini, a sesame seed puree).

2–3 vegetables grown above ground with one vegetable grown be-low ground.

2–4 ounces red wine with brown bread in the late afternoon, 3–4 times a week, is a blood and body builder.

Gelatin with raw vegetables or fruit.

Orange juice with 1–2 tablespoons lemon juice. Grapefruit juice with 1–2 tablespoons lime juice. (Adding lemon/lime balances the ef-fect of hybridization of citrus.)

Acid/Alkaline Balance

THE pH BALANCE

The pH is measured on a scale from 0 to 14. Anything above 7 is alkaline, and anything below 7 is acid.

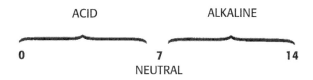

ACID   ALKALINE

0   7   14

NEUTRAL

For optimal health, the pH of the blood should be 7.4. The saliva pH should be mainly alkaline, and the urine pH should be on the acid side. In order to maintain this balance, the ideal ratio of food that we eat every day should be 80% alkaline and 20% acid. However, if en-gaging in heavy, physical labor, the ratio can be 70/30, for exercise burns up acids. Since our body is a machine that constantly makes acid waste products, it is very important that a diet be followed that consists mainly of alkaline fruits and vegetables.

Alkaline Foods	Acid Foods
• Fruits (except cranberries, plums, prunes)	• Cranberries, plums, prunes
	• Dried beans
• Vegetables (except dried beans)	• All other nuts
• Almonds, brazil nuts	• Egg whites, whole eggs
• Egg yolks	• All grains and flour products (except millet and buckwheat)
• Millet, buckwheat	
	• Pasteurized milk products
• Raw milk products	
	• Sugar and other sweeteners (except honey)
• Honey	
• Seeds (sesame, pumpkin, sunflower)	• Animal protein (meat, fish, fowl)
	• Prescription drugs
	• Coffee, tea, sodas

When the diet is too acidic, digestion suffers, the eliminations decline, and the cells become toxic. We then experience lethargy, fatigue, depression, joint pain, stiff muscles, and other symptoms of toxicity, which sets us up for colds and chronic illness.

To swing in the other direction and become overly alkaline is even more harmful, according to Cayce. When this happens, we may feel anxious, spacey, excited, or experience muscle spasms. The pH can quickly change whenever there is stress or negative emotions, no matter how well-balanced the diet has been.

HOW TO MONITOR THE pH

The pH of the saliva or urine can *easily* be checked with litmus or nitrazine paper.

Saliva

Since eating and drinking will affect the pH results for several hours, the optimal time for testing is before breakfast or just before dinner. The normal range is 6.8 to 7.5.

Urine

Urine should be collected in a clean, glass bottle over a 24–hour period, and then tested. Discard the first morning urine; then, begin collecting with the next urination, and continue through the first morning urine of the next day. (Since the pH changes throughout the day, collecting the urine over a 24–hour period gives a more accurate picture of the alkaline/acid balance of the body. And because the first urination of the day contains bacteria and other waste cleared from the body during the night, it is better to add it to the bottle at the end of the 24 hours, rather than at the beginning.) The normal pH range for urine is 6.3 to 7.

How to Test

Litmus paper: Take one strip, and wet it with saliva or urine.

Results: Blue will indicate alkalinity; pink will indicate acidity.

Nitrazine paper: Tear off a one–inch strip, and wet it with saliva or urine. Wait 10–15 seconds, and compare it with the color chart on the dispenser.

Results: Blue will indicate alkaline, and green to yellow will indicate acidity.

Cayce suggested that the pH be monitored in the morning, once a week. Citrus fruit or juice can then be taken at breakfast if the saliva pH is below 6.8 or the urine pH is below 6.3. He also gave a very unusual method to reduce acidity: Several people were told to suck the juice of half a lemon, followed by one to two glasses of water. Let 10-15 minutes go by (perhaps taking a walk). Then, after adding a pinch of salt to the other half of the lemon, suck the juice, followed by four to six more glasses of water.

Summary

1) Each person must choose the diet that feels right by using common sense and paying attention to what agrees and disagrees with one's system.

2) Other factors besides taste, appearance, and texture affect our digestion.

3) Improper food combining and foods that are difficult to digest stress the entire digestion process.

4) An abundance of fruits and vegetables gives the colon much needed fiber, and stimulates the eliminations.

5) For optimal health with a blood pH of 7.4, our daily food intake should be 80% alkaline and 20% acid.

6) The pH can be checked weekly with litmus or nitrazine paper, so that the diet can be adjusted accordingly.

SIX

Fasting

But nature's storehouse, (thine own body) may be induced to create every influence necessary for bringing greater and better and nearer normal conditions, if the hindrances are removed.

1309-1

Guidelines

Fasting is a time-honored way of treating illness and detoxifying the body from any overindulgent or detrimental eating patterns. It is also a spiritual discipline; as the spiritual, mental, and emotional levels become aligned, the mind becomes clearer, the vital force of the body is recharged, and a higher level of attunement with the Divine within may be reached. True fasting, Edgar Cayce expressed, is a way for us to cast out our lower ego self and replace it with our Higher Self: "as Thou, O Lord, seest fit" (295-6).

There are many ways to fast. The appropriate choice depends upon one's age, physical health, stress, toxicity, and diet patterns. It is best to begin slowly with either freshly juiced fruits or vegetables, or one of Cayce's mono fruit diets that will permit the body to detoxify while still receiving adequate nutrients. One should be cautious when on a more severe water or dry fast, for toxins are heavily released at this time.

Fasting should not be undertaken if you have a serious illness, hypoglycemia, cannot gain weight easily, or if you are pregnant or nursing a baby. It is also not recommended for children.

Fasting can make you feel spacey, so it is wise to plan ahead for a time when your work schedule is not too demanding or when you will have time off, depending, of course, on the nature of your particular occupation. Driving or operating dangerous machinery, etc., is not advisable at this time. It is important to rest, not overdo, and to defer social plans.

Healing Crisis

During a fast, the four major organs of elimination work overtime to purge the accumulation of dross in the system. If these organs are unable to keep up with the demand, what is termed a "healing crisis" may occur, and one or more of the following conditions may manifest: foul breath, a coated tongue, increased body odor, joint pain, muscle aches, nausea, headaches, foul-smelling stools, crusted eyes in the morning, or a runny nose, as old mucus is eliminated. Many people stop fasting when they feel this way because they erroneously think that the fast is making them ill. What is actually happening, however, is that the cells are throwing off toxins faster than the eliminating channels can handle them, and the toxins then migrate to other areas, such as the joints, the lungs, or the muscles, etc., where they cause further problems.

Hydrotherapy

It is absolutely necessary to exercise and cleanse the body with hydrotherapy beginning with the first day of any fast. The organs of elimination need this extra help in order to cope with the excessive amount of toxins being released. If they can keep up with the demand, you will feel lighter and more energized without any uncomfortable symptoms.

Hydrotherapy, or water therapy, is an ancient healing modality for maintaining health and preventing illness. During a fast, the most supportive hydrotherapies are colonics, enemas, Epsom salts baths, steam/ fume baths, saunas, and the drinking of pure water.

If colonics are available, one should be taken on the first day of a two- to five-day fast, followed by a two-quart enema on each succeeding day. If a fast lasts from 5-14 days, two to three colonics should be taken, with enemas every two to three days in between. If the fast is to exceed 14 days, it should be monitored by a health care professional.

Epsom salts baths, saunas, and steam/fume baths increase perspiration and eliminate excess toxins through the skin. They should be avoided when one has high blood pressure, heart, or kidney problems.

Daily brushing of the skin with a natural-bristle bath brush or a loofah removes any dead skin cells and allows the pores to sweat more effectively.

EPSOM SALTS BATH

- Add 1 cup Epsom salts per 60 pounds body weight to 6 inches of 102° bath water.
- Stir thoroughly to dissolve the salts.
- Get into the tub and continue to fill with water as the temperature rises to 106°.
- Soak for 15-20 minutes.
- Stop at any time if you feel uncomfortable, overheated, or lightheaded.
- Afterwards, wrap up in a towel, lie down, and continue to sweat for 30 minutes.
- Follow with a shower in tepid to cool water. Do not use soap, which clogs the pores and inhibits the release of toxins.

Another way to increase perspiration is to have a steam bath in a sweat cabinet. The design of the cabinet, which encases the body up to the neck, allows the head to be free of the higher temperatures inside the cabinet. Ice-cold cloths may easily be placed on the forehead and the base of the neck to constrict the blood vessels and prevent headaches. Cayce often recommended that essential oils and other sub-stances be vaporized as a fume to stimulate the removal of toxins through the skin and lungs. Atomidine, pine needle oil, wintergreen, and witch hazel are commonly used.

The kidneys and urinary tract are flushed and cleansed by drinking six to eight glasses of pure water each day. Cayce, you must realize, said that water should be gently sipped, then actually chewed three to four times, in order to mingle with the secretions of the glands in the mouth before being swallowed.

Deep breathing and moderate exercise, such as walking—which Cayce declared *the* best overall exercise for the body—detoxify the lungs. Massage is also very beneficial in stimulating the blood and lymph circulation to rid the body of toxins and fatigue poisons.

Preparation for a Fast

One should ease into a fast gradually by taking a few days to wean oneself of dairy, grain, and animal products. Organic fruits and veg-etables are preferable, but if only commercial produce is available, the pesticides may be removed from the skin with a bleach bath. To do so, add one tablespoon bleach to one gallon water, soak 15 minutes, then rinse off.

Although fasting may be undertaken at any time, fresh fruits are more plentiful in the spring, summer, and fall. Ideally, fasting should be done when a fruit is at its peak of life force energy. An apple diet in May, for example, would not be as beneficial as an orange fast in May because the apples have been in cold storage for several months. When fruits and vegetables are in season and locally grown, they are vibrationally more compatible with the body.

Cayce's Three Fruit Fasts

Cayce suggested three types of mono fruit diets, a fast in which only one kind of raw fruit is eaten for the duration of the fast. Cayce de-clared that the 3-day apple diet, his most popular, would "cleanse all toxic forces from any system!" (820–2). However, it is often necessary that the fast be repeated to become really effective. In this diet, no fewer than five jennetting apples (an early variety), such as Jonathan, Delicious, Oregon Red, or Arkansas Black, are to be eaten throughout each day. (Jennetting apples were also called "sheepnose" because of the pattern of five protuberances on the bottom, which distinguishes them from the round-bottomed varieties such as Gala or Granny Smith.) The apples should be in season, well-ripened, and each bite thoroughly masticated 4–20 times.

Cayce was very wise in recommending apples, for they contain a hydrophilic fruit pectin that acts as a bactericide as it sweeps through the intestinal tract, absorbing and removing toxins. It also inhibits the growth of many putrefactive bacteria. He further mentions that apples cleanse not only the liver and kidneys, but also the entire system.

Perhaps it is this cleansing property that accounts for Cayce's recommendation that apples be eaten alone—not in combination with other foods—for they are apparently hard to digest and assimilate otherwise. This is not the case when they are cooked, but for fasting purposes use only the raw fruit.

The grape diet is mentioned only a few times in the readings. In this diet, quantities of local, purple Concord grapes with the seeds removed are eaten throughout a four-day period. Joanna Brandt, author of *The Grape Cure*, states that grapes break up unhealthy tissue and dissolve hardened mucus that has adhered to the intestinal wall. As the blood is purified on a grape fast, the system is drained of poisons, allowing the cells to rebuild and rejuvenate. Ms. Brandt was personally healed of cancer after nine years of searching for a fast that would permanently destroy her tumor. Once she discovered the use of grapes, she was cured.

If oranges are preferred, any amount may be eaten throughout each day for five days. One woman was advised to eat about a dozen a day; otherwise, the amount is not specified.

On the last evening of each of the three fasts, olive oil is recommended at bedtime to aid the body's removal of residual, hard fecal matter. The amount of olive oil advised varies from two teaspoonfuls to one-half teacup, but it is best to begin with two teaspoonfuls to make sure the oil is well-tolerated.

The drinking of coffee or tea may be continued throughout the fast for those who are accustomed to it, so long as no cream, milk, or sugar is added. Although Cayce categorized coffee as a food for the body, caffeine at times throws off poisons when it remains in the colon, and this dross needs to be eliminated. If you are considering giving up coffee or tea altogether, this may be a good time to do so.

Breaking a fast and easing back into eating again may be more challenging than the actual period of fasting. The digestive system, having been shut down, must now be slowly and carefully started up again in order to fully benefit from the fast. Grains and animal protein should be reintroduced slowly to avoid stressing the body. This is a very good time to become aware of old habits, and begin to develop new, more healthy eating patterns.

The following charts outline general guidelines for fasting and cleansing with Cayce's three mono diets.

HOW TO FAST

Apples	Grapes	Oranges
DAY ONE		
A minimum of 5 Delicious apples	Handful of Concord grapes every 2-3 hours	Oranges, as desired
6-8 glasses purified water	6-8 glasses purified water	6-8 glasses purified water
Colonic	Colonic	Colonic
Brisk 30-minute walk	Brisk 30-minute walk	Brisk 30-minute walk
DAY TWO		
5+ apples	Grapes every 2-3 hours	Oranges as desired
6-8 glasses purified water	6-8 glasses purified water	6-8 glasses purified water
Dry skin brush, then steam/fume followed by a massage	Dry skin brush, then steam/fume followed by a massage	Dry skin brush, then steam/fume followed by a massage
Enema	Enema	Enema
DAY THREE		
5+ apples	Grapes every 2-3 hours	Oranges as desired
6-8 glasses purified water	6-8 glasses purified water	6-8 glasses purified water
Epsom salts bath	Epsom salts bath	Epsom salts bath
30-minute walk	30-minute walk	30-minute walk
Enema	Enema	Enema
2 teaspoons olive oil at bedtime		
END OF FAST		

Apples	Grapes	Oranges
DAY FOUR		
Expand to other fruits (no melons, bananas, or raw apples) 6-8 glasses purified water 30-minute walk Enema, only if feeling toxic	Handful grapes every 2-3 hours 6-8 glasses purified water 30-minute walk Dry skin brush, then steam/fume afterwards Enema 2 teaspoons olive oil at bedtime **END OF FAST**	Oranges, as desired 6-8 glasses purified water 30-minute walk Dry skin brush, then steam/fume afterwards Enema

DAY FIVE		
Breakfast: Fruit 9-11 a.m.: 3 glasses purified water Lunch: Raw vegetable salad with olive oil/lemon juice 3-5 p.m.: 3 glasses purified water Supper: Raw or steamed vegetables	Expand to other fruits (no melons, bananas or raw apples) 6-8 glasses purified water 30-minute walk Enema, only if feeling toxic	Oranges, as desired 6-8 glasses purified water Epsom salts bath 30-minute walk Enema 2 teaspoons olive oil at bedtime **END OF FAST**

	Apples	Grapes	Oranges
DAY SIX			
	Breakfast: Fruit 9-11 a.m.: 3 glasses purified water Lunch: Raw vegetable salad with olive oil or lemon juice 3-5 p.m.: 3 glasses purified water Supper: Protein: animal or grain+bean, vegetables: 2-3 above-ground 1 below-ground	Breakfast: Fruit 9-11 a.m.: 3 glasses purified water Lunch: Raw vegetable salad with olive oil or lemon juice 3-5 p.m.: 3 glasses purified water Supper: Raw or steamed vegetables	Expand to other fruits (no melons, bananas or raw apples) 6-8 glasses purified water 30-minute walk Enema, only if feeling toxic

DAY SEVEN			
		Breakfast: Fruit 9-11 a.m.: 3 glasses purified water Lunch: Raw vegetable salad with olive oil or lemon juice 3-5 p.m.: 3 glasses purified water Supper: Protein: animal or grain+bean, vegetables: 2-3 above-ground 1 below-ground	Breakfast: Fruit 9-11 a.m.: 3 glasses purified water Lunch: Raw vegetable salad with olive oil or lemon juice 3-5 p.m.: 3 glasses purified water Supper: Raw or steamed vegetables

DAY EIGHT			
			Same as Grapes, Day 7

Summary

1) Periodic fasting improves the quality of one's health and, as a con-sequence, heightens our awareness of the indwelling life force.

2) Colon cleansing and other hydrotherapies are absolutely neces-sary during a fast to prevent a healing crisis.

3) Preparing for a fast, and gradually resuming a normal eating pat-tern *after* a fast, may be more challenging than the fast itself.

4) Edgar Cayce gave us three mono fruit diets to choose from: three days of Jonathan variety or Delicious apples, four days of Concord grapes, or five days of oranges.

" . . . what we think and what we eat—combined together— make what we are; physically and mentally." 288-38

Edgar Cayce Basic Diet

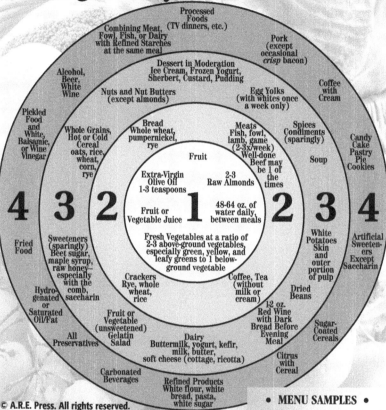

DIRECTIONS

Circle 1: Alkaline food: 80% of your daily intake—four or five servings.

Circle 2: Acid food: 20% of your daily intake.

Circle 3: Three times a week.

Circle 4: Avoid these foods.

- Eat local produce whenever possible—local organic would be best of all!

Edgar Cayce's A.R.E.® (Association for Research and Enlightenment, Inc.), 215 67th Street, Virginia Beach, VA 23451-2061. Phone (757) 428-3588; 1-800-333-4499 Web site: EdgarCayce.org

Edgar Cayce Readings ©1971, 1993-2007 by the Edgar Cayce Foundation. All Rights Reserved.

The information contained in the Edgar Cayce readings should not be regarded as a guide to self-diagnosis or self-treatment. The cooperation of a qualified health care professional is essential if one wishes to apply the principles and techniques described in the readings.

• MENU SAMPLES •

- BREAKFAST -
Cereal with milk and berries *or*
Scrambled or coddled eggs with toast (whole wheat, rye, pumpernickel) *or*
Fruit (citrus, melons alone)

- LUNCH -
Raw salad (especially leaf lettuce, celery, carrots) with olive oil dressing and/or vegetable soup, whole grain bread, or crackers

- DINNER -
Fish, fowl, lamb, beef well-done
Cooked vegetables (2-3 above ground to 1 below ground)
Dessert (in moderation)

SEVEN

Some Case Histories

. . . it is as necessary to keep the body coordinating and clean as it is to keep the mental attitude right as well as the correct spiritual purposes and desires and, most of all, keep all three consistently; and don't be one thing in one way and another in another way . . . Do right yourself physically, mentally and spiritually and the best will come to you.   5203-1

Hypertension/High Blood Pressure

Normal blood pressure is the force of blood exerted against the arterial blood vessel wall. It changes continually throughout the day in response to food, emotion, exercise, breathing, and stress. Hypertension, or high blood pressure, is a chronic elevation of pressure; however, there is some disagreement as to the guidelines for measuring it. The World Health Organization states that anything over 140/90 should be treated, whereas the American Heart Association says that anything over 160/90 should be the criterion for treating adults over 40 years of age.

Approximately 25 people requested a reading for this problem, including Edgar Cayce himself, who suffered from it for two years following surgery for appendicitis. In every case, the basic cause is attributed to sluggish eliminations, excess toxins, and spinal misalignments. *All* those who followed the advice given in their readings were cured, as was Cayce.

There is a fascinating exchange of letters between Cayce and a Mr. 4345 who—although he had consulted doctors and made various dietary changes had been suffering from high blood pressure without any relief for years. His reading on August 9, 1932, indicates that years of constipation had caused areas in the ascending and transverse colon to dilate, resulting in a toxic build-up not only in the colon, but throughout his whole system. Toxins put pressure on the blood, heart, liver, kidneys, and digestion and, as a result, the venous and arterial circulation were not working together properly. His reading paints a very clear picture of the domino effect that happens when the colon becomes congested with toxic build-up. (See the "Toxic Build-Up" section in Chapter Four and the diagram on page 73.)

The suggested treatment was to have four to six colon irrigations, at the rate of one every two weeks, along with two general osteopathic manipulations each week. The spinal adjustments were to be administered to stimulate the cerebrospinal and autonomic centers in the neck and upper back regions. Such an injunction—to have four to six colonics and as many as two dozen osteopathic adjustments, followed by routine maintenance colonics to prevent the dilation from recurring—required quite a commitment in both time and money.

Cayce took a personal interest in this case, and enclosed the following letter, relating that he had also been cured by following similar guidance from his own reading.

My Dear Mr. 4345,
. . . Our experience through the years has been that such treatments [osteopathic adjustments and colonics] are most successful in reducing pressure, when they are kept for a sufficient length of time to overcome the disorder, so as to prevent a return. Following an operation for myself some years ago I had high blood pressure, which was very annoying for two years. Then in

DOMINO EFFECT OF TOXINS
ON HIGH BLOOD PRESSURE
(4345-1)

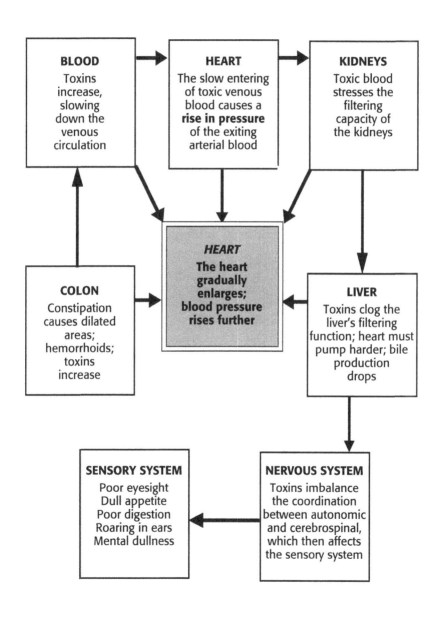

BLOOD
Toxins increase, slowing down the venous circulation

HEART
The slow entering of toxic venous blood causes a **rise in pressure** of the exiting arterial blood

KIDNEYS
Toxic blood stresses the filtering capacity of the kidneys

HEART
The heart gradually enlarges; blood pressure rises further

COLON
Constipation causes dilated areas; hemorrhoids; toxins increase

LIVER
Toxins clog the liver's filtering function; heart must pump harder; bile production drops

SENSORY SYSTEM
Poor eyesight
Dull appetite
Poor digestion
Roaring in ears
Mental dullness

NERVOUS SYSTEM
Toxins imbalance the coordination between autonomic and cerebrospinal, which then affects the sensory system

a reading treatments similar to yours were suggested for me, and I had the opportunity to have them carried out properly. Since then I have never suffered with the condition. That is my own personal experience. Quite a number of cases similar we have had during the years, and most remarkable results have been obtained from following the treatments outlined. I hope such will be true in your case.

I trust you will let us hear from you from time to time, and if there is anything we can do to be of service please know that we are only too glad to try.

Two months later, the man wrote to complain that he had "complied with the suggestions exactly . . . but do not find any change." In fact, his blood pressure was a little higher. Cayce replied that he was very surprised to hear this, as it had never happened when the directions were followed exactly as given.

He immediately offered a check reading, which said that *massages* had been taken *instead* of osteopathy. The colonics had indeed relieved the pressures and toxicity in the colon, but the massages had neither relieved nor corrected the pressures along the spine. Osteopathy, of course, is very different from Swedish massage. It helps maintain a balance between the autonomic and cerebrospinal nervous systems, and increases circulation to produce drainage. A form of osteopathic massage relieves muscle tension and impingements on spinal nerves that, in turn, help realign the vertebrae.

The reading said Mr. 4345 was to repeat the colonics and have osteopathic adjustments specifically in the upper to middle dorsals (now called thoracics) and throughout the cervical area. Cayce told him that if he followed the directions and did everything properly that it *"will not fail."*

Out of curiosity, Cayce again wrote to the man four months later to see what was happening. A brief reply simply said he had complied with the directions and, as a result, his blood pressure was down. His general health had apparently also improved.

In 1940, a 51-year-old woman (780-10) wanted to know if her blood pressure was any cause for alarm. She ran a rooming house and was raising four children while her salesman husband was away most of the time. She had been in fairly good health, but had gradually become obese over the years, and was now experiencing some heart and high blood pressure problems. Her reading explained that the heart and blood pressure work in coordination with each other and, consequently, her condition was very serious. She was advised to have colonics and osteopathy—the colonics to remove the cause, which was pressure in the colon, and the osteopathy to correct the incoordination between the heart and the blood pressure.

Several months later, her husband reported that she had lost weight and was doing just fine. However, in two years she had relapsed with her diet, and Cayce again warned her to keep the colon cleansed, for a fullness in the colon had developed and her blood pressure was borderline. She continued to have blood pressure and weight problems until her death in 1951.

Heart Problems

People often inquired about the condition of their heart only to learn, surprisingly, that it was the unhealthy condition of the colon that was adversely affecting the heart's normal functioning. A 49-year-old man (1057), for example, wanted to know what caused his suspected heart attack. Cayce informed him that he had not had a heart attack; an engorgement in the colon had produced an increase in pressure in the circulation, adversely affecting nerves and causing heart pain.

Although the idea that a pathological condition in the colon can directly affect the heart may seem farfetched, Cayce indeed found that engorged areas in the colon cause bothersome symptoms of dizziness, shortness of breath, irregular pulse, and even heart pain. Often, as in the case just mentioned, the physical reading would find no organic heart disease present, and once the colon problems were cleared up— through colonic irrigations and other specific suggestions—aberrant heart symptoms would disappear. But he did warn that if the colon condition were untended, the heart would eventually develop a diseased state. It makes one wonder how much heart disease could be prevented with proper colon care. In the few cases involving individuals already on heart medication at the time their readings were requested, Cayce said the heart medicine could be gradually decreased *under a doctor's supervision if* the guidance given in the reading were followed.

Let me share two further cases from the readings. A 70-year-old man (1772-2) was told to have one or two good colonic irrigations to remove the mucus that was causing congestion and pressure on the circulation—not only to the heart, but to the lungs and kidneys as well. How simple: cleansing the colon would allow these organs to function more normally and to avoid further dysfunction.

A 56-year-old man (370-7) was very concerned about heart palpitations and chest pains, wanting to know if he had done anything to cause this condition. He became so anxious he couldn't sleep at night. Fortunately, his condition turned out to be much less alarming than he had anticipated. Cayce reassured him that the heart condition was due to nervous tension and a toxic build-up caused by poor eliminations. The advice was short and direct: "The removal of the poisons and the use of the colonics will correct this." In one sense, Mr. 370's concern over feeling responsible for his symptoms *was* truly valid, for one's lifestyle, emotions, and eating patterns all affect the eliminations.

Prostatitis

Colon cleansing is a major factor in the prevention of illness. In his book, *The Edgar Cayce Handbook for Health through Drugless Therapy*, Dr. Harold J. Reilly says that he and Cayce had always advised colonics, sitz baths, and breach-beating (discussed later in the chapter) as a protection from and a treatment for prostatitis, or inflammation of the prostate gland. The prostate often becomes not only enlarged and infected, but can cause difficulty with urination as well. Colonics help to remove toxins from the prostate that contribute to the inflammation and infection.

A 61-year-old man (3570) was told that the lack of peristaltic movement in his colon was putting pressure on his prostate gland. He was told to have an occasional colonic irrigation. Dr. Reilly recalls Cayce's belief that "a man who took a colonic every month would never have this trouble common to aging males" (p. 478, large paperback edition).

Sitz baths are an extremely effective hydrotherapy for stimulating circulation to pelvic organs and reducing swelling and inflammation of the prostate. The addition to the bathwater of one cup Epsom salts per 60 pounds body weight further stimulates the detoxification effect by removing toxins through the skin. One sits waist deep—with the feet *out of the water*—in 100° to 106° water for 10-15 minutes. These baths may be taken three to four times a week in an acute situation, or one to two times a month as a maintenance routine. Alternating the temperature from hot to cold three times has an even more stimulating effect. The bath should always begin hot (100°-106°) for two to four minutes and end cold (45°-65°) for 30 seconds.

Breach-beating is a form of tapotement or percussion massage in which the fists alternately strike the buttocks with a series of rapid, rhythmic movements. This vibrates the prostate gland and increases circulation to the area. It can be done by oneself or by a massage therapist.

A 58-year-old man (1196) received 17 readings over a seven-year period for poor eliminations, an inflamed prostate, liver/gallbladder problems, and rheumatism. His main complaints were excessive gas, constipation, and pain in his lower abdomen, hips, legs, and back. He also informed Cayce of his spastic colon, and that his tongue was always heavily coated (a sign of constipation).

The reading disclosed a condition of toxemia caused by poor eliminations that had congested his liver, impaired the hepatic circulation between the liver and kidneys, and created a weakness in the prostate. The excessive amount of toxins in his body was causing the rheumatism in his hips, legs, and back, and the weakened condition of the prostate was adversely affecting his lower abdomen.

Cayce said he should consider sugar, fats, and fried foods taboo, as they created a hardship on his liver and pancreas. The fats and toxins also upset his digestion and caused gas. Enemas, using a soft rectal tube, were advised to reverse the engorgement in the descending colon, thereby stimulating better eliminations. Osteopathy was recommended to relieve pressures and increase the circulation to spinal nerves affecting the alimentary canal. He was also told to drink six to eight glasses of water a day to flush his kidneys.

He did not fully carry out the suggestions given, and his next reading again stressed the importance of following *all* of the guidance given. Cayce explained that certain of the recommendations had been given to awaken and arouse toxins, and that if the toxins were not eliminated, they would cause congestion in other areas. He then told Mr. 1196 to "either *accept* the suggestions *as* given, or to *reject* them entirely!"

Several readings later, Mr. 1196-12 was asking what made him sleepy too early at night and what caused his "extreme inward nervousness." Cayce replied that this was due to toxic forces. The dietary suggestions had not been followed, and now his emotions were making matters worse. According to the reading, his hatred, animosity, and anxiety had created poisons that were not easily eliminated. Together, his negative emotions and the inability to stay away from fats, grease, and fried foods created an acute gallbladder problem and an inflamed, irritated prostate.

He was told to have consistent treatments, three times a week, with the Elliot machine (which is no longer manufactured). It was a motor-driven pump with gauges and valves that controlled the pressure and temperature, and a container to heat water. A rubber applicator was inserted into the rectum and gradually filled with hot water to produce a mechanical distention of three to four pounds of pressure. This was very effective in reducing the swelling and inflammation in the prostate gland.

Another method of treating prostatitis was shortwave diathermy, which is still in use today. A lamp or a machine with a heating pad is used to produce deep heat in the tissues. In Cayce's day, it was preferred by many doctors over the Elliot machine because it was more convenient to use.

Unfortunately, the guidance given to Mr. 1196 was apparently never fully carried out, and his condition deteriorated over the years. In 1943, he told Cayce that he had felt much better after his first reading, but had to drop everything when his wife became ill and could no longer help him.

The Common Cold

Whenever you are coming down with a cold, the readings say to have a colonic. I know from my own experience that this helps, especially if initiated at the first sign of a runny nose or sore throat. I never knew why this was effective until I read Dr. Bieler's explanation, in *Food Is Your Best Medicine,* that "there is always a toxic state before a cold" (p. 167).

There are several factors, according to Cayce, that predispose one towards "catching" a cold: exhaustion, toxicity, wet feet, and experiencing a cold draft about the body. When the level of toxins becomes too high for the liver, kidneys, and colon to handle, the next organ to be affected is the thyroid gland, which is in charge of the mucous membranes. A runny nose is the body's way of releasing or removing toxins, and gives us the message that we need to rest and cleanse. If a colonic or enema is taken at the *earliest* signs, the toxin level quickly drops, and the cold may disappear completely. Even if several hours have elapsed before the colonic is taken, the intensity of the cold may still be significantly lessened. If a full-blown cold does develop, however, Dr. Bieler adds that germs then gather to take advantage of the situation, and eat the toxic wastes that follow inflammation.

Our level of toxicity can rise slowly over several months, or it can increase suddenly with intense negative emotions, such as when we lose our temper, for anger literally poisons the system. Cayce called anger a disease of the mind caused by frustration and fear. The overload of adrenalin slows down the blood, clogs the liver, upsets the kidneys, and blocks the flow of blood to the eliminating channels. A woman once came to me for a colonic because she had come down with a severe cold just 24 hours after being extremely angry with her husband. She said she intuitively knew that the cold was somehow related to the anger, for she felt polluted by having lost her emotional control.

When we are exposed to someone who has a cold, we will not catch it if our blood pH is slightly alkaline, for the cold virus cannot live in an alkaline environment. At the first sign of a cold, a very effective Cayce method to quickly alkalinize is to drink 48 ounces of orange juice mixed with the juice of two fresh lemons during a 30-minute period. The key to success is to drink it at the earliest symptoms. The pH turns alkaline in four to five hours, as indicated by a subtle yet perceptible shift in the throat—a smooth feeling, if you will—and the cold magically disappears. If the symptoms return in a day or two, the orange juice procedure may be repeated. This recurrence seems to happen when the level of toxins is still high, and the thyroid again gets the signal to detoxify. A recurrence is less likely to happen if the colon is cleansed at the same time.

Although oranges and lemons are known to be acid fruits, they are alkaline-reacting in the body. The first oranges of the season are the richest in vitamin C and minerals, and fully-ripened ones are the most alkaline-reacting. Oranges are very good for sluggish eliminations, though some individuals will experience a temporary diarrhea from drinking the 48 ounces of juice in 30 minutes.

Summary

1) High blood pressure was cured for many people, including Cayce, by following the advice given in their readings to have colonics and osteopathic treatments.

2) Non-organic heart problems are often directly related to an engorged condition of the colon.

3) Dr. Reilly and Cayce always advised colonics, sitz baths, and breach-beating for prostatitis.

4) Cayce prescribed a monthly colonic to prevent prostate trouble.

5) There is always a toxic state prior to a cold. Colonics and an orange juice regimen will detoxify and alkalinize the system quickly so that the cold will go away.

EIGHT

Colon Hydrotherapy

Q. How often should hydrotherapy be given?
A. Dependent upon the general conditions. Whenever there is a sluggishness, the feeling of heaviness, oversleepiness, the tendency for an achy, draggy feeling, then have the treatments.

This does not mean that merely because there is the daily activity of the alimentary canal there is no need for flushing the system. But whenever there is the feeling of sluggishness, have the treatments. It'll pick the body up. For there is a need for such treatments when the condition of the body becomes drugged because of absorption of poisons through [the] alimentary canal or colon, sluggishness of liver or kidneys, and there is the lack of coordination with the cerebrospinal and sympathetic [autonomic] blood supply and nerves. For the hydrotherapy and massage are preventive as well as curative measures. For the cleansing of the system allows the body-forces themselves to function normally, and thus eliminate poisons, congestions, and conditions that would become acute through the body. 257-254

Enema/Fountain Syringe

At home, a water enema is the simplest way to irrigate the colon to temporarily relieve constipation or to remove toxins, especially during a fast. The water usually reaches only the sigmoid and descending colon during this procedure. If the colon is already constipated, it may be somewhat uncomfortable.

Although enemas are not meant to be taken on a regular basis as a substitute for normal eliminations, over 1,000 readings suggested that they be used until the underlying cause of constipation could be corrected. Cayce also recommended using antiseptics such as salt/baking soda and Glyco-Thymoline, for enemas as well as colonics, to purify the system.

A kit may be purchased from any pharmacy and consists of a two-quart rubber bag, a four-foot piece of tubing with a clamp, a two-and-a-half-inch enema nozzle, and a five-inch douche nozzle. (Carefully read the enclosed directions from the kit you will be using, but make sure you always lie on your left side during the enema procedure, no matter what the kit says.)

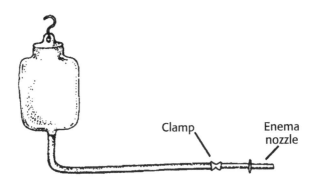

ENEMA SET-UP

1) Close the clamp on the 4-foot piece of tubing and attach the shorter enema nozzle.

2) Fill the bag with body-temperature water (around 98–99°). If you do not have a thermometer, place some water on your wrist. It should feel neutral (neither hot nor cold).

3) First bag: thoroughly dissolve 1 heaping teaspoon of salt and 1 level teaspoon baking soda in ½ cup water. Add this mixture to the bag and stir well.

4) Open the clamp and let water run through the tubing to remove any air, then reclamp.

5) Lubricate the nozzle with castor oil or vaseline.

6) Hang the bag on the bathroom doorknob. (However, if someone can assist you, then lie on a bed as the assistant holds the bag no higher than 18 inches above you.)

7) Lie on your left side on the bathroom floor; do *not* sit on the toilet.

8) Gently insert the lubricated tip into the rectum.

9) Open the clamp slowly. If you have a feeling of fullness at any time, try closing the clamp, waiting 5-10 seconds and then unclamping. The colon does not like to be rushed, and may be able to be filled with more water this way.

10) Although ideally you should be able to take almost all the water, the colon may only be able to accept ¼ or ½ of the bag at this time.

11) When you feel full, re-clamp, remove the nozzle, and sit on the toilet to expel the water.

12) Empty any leftover solution, rinse the bag and tubing, and re-clamp.

13) Second bag: refill with body-temperature water, add 2 tablespoons Glyco-Thymoline, and stir well.

14) Repeat steps 4 through 9, taking in as much water as possible.

15) Re-clamp, remove the nozzle, and expel the water into the toilet.

16) When done, wash the nozzle with a germicidal solution, and hang the bag to dry before storage.

There are several other kinds of enemas: coffee, medicated, oil retention, and a three-stage.

COFFEE ENEMA

The coffee solution is meant to be retained in the colon for a short time to help detoxify the liver.

In a saucepan, add 3 tablespoons ground coffee to 1 quart water. Boil for 3 minutes, then simmer for 20 minutes.

For the enema, strain the coffee and use at body temperature.

Slowly and gradually—so that there will not be the urge to evacuate—let the solution run into the colon.

Retain the liquid for 15–30 minutes, and then expel in the toilet.

MEDICATED ENEMA

This comes in a 4½ ounce bottle with its own tip and may be purchased from any pharmacy. It contains sodium phosphate, which pulls water from the mucous membranes of the rectum and stimulates an evacuation.

OIL RETENTION ENEMA

This also comes in a 4½ ounce bottle with its own tip, and contains mineral oil, which is helpful in softening hard, impacted fecal matter in the rectum. The liquid should be retained for 30 minutes before being expelled, followed by a 2–quart water enema.

THREE-STAGE ENEMA

If a colonic was not available when fasting, Dr. Reilly would suggest a three–stage enema to get results more comparable to a colonic.

First bag: Thoroughly dissolve 1 heaping teaspoon salt and 1 level teaspoon baking soda in ½ cup water. Stir well, and add to 2–quart enema bag filled with warm water. Lie on your left side.

Second bag: Repeat above, but kneel in a knee–chest position.

Third bag: Add 2 tablespoons Glyco–Thymoline to the bag filled with warm water, and lie on your *right* side.

COLON TUBE (HIGH ENEMA)

The earlier readings mention colon tubes more frequently than those given in the 1940s, possibly because such tubes were more difficult to obtain in wartime, or perhaps colonics were not always available. Nevertheless, people often asked if their colonic could be done at home. Sometimes Cayce responded that the first two or three colonics should be given professionally, and then a colon tube could be used at home. It reaches the bend on the left side of the colon (the splenic flexure), thus enabling the water to be more effective in stimulating peristalsis in the transverse and ascending colon.

The colon tube is available from a medical supply house or a pharmacy that carries such home health supplies as wheelchairs, crutches, etc. The length should be 30 inches (76.2 cm) with a diameter of 16–32 Fr. (French).

To use, simply slip the open end of the tube over the enema nozzle, and follow the directions for "Enema Set-up," page 84, with the following changes:

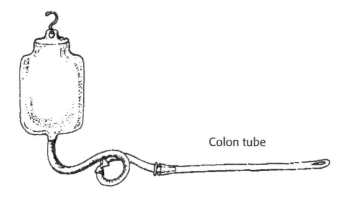

Colon tube

Lubricate ¾ of the length with castor oil or vaseline.

Insert the tube slowly and gently as far as possible, but *do not force.* If any resistance is felt, pull the tube back a few inches and gently try again.

Cayce cautioned against trying to cleanse the whole colon at one time when first using a colon tube, and to gradually insert it higher and higher over several irrigations. One person was told to alternate an enema with the colon tube to prevent its being overused.

COLEMA

Dr. Bernard Jensen, in *Tissue Cleansing Through Bowel Management*, calls the colema a special kind of high enema. It is used two or even three times a day in conjunction with his cleansing program. It tones up the bowel wall, and encourages normal peristalsis without distending the colon. A patented colema board—approximately 45 x 15 inches—is used. One end rests on a chair or stool, and the other end has a hole and splash board that goes over the toilet. A five-gallon bucket that holds the water is placed two or three feet above the board. And although the colema is called a high enema, the tubing is inserted only 2–3 inches into the rectum.

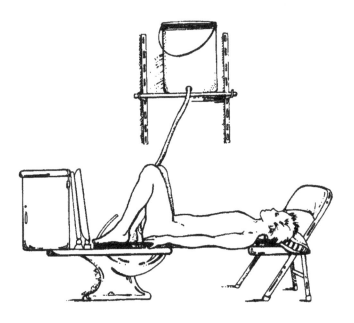

One advantage of this method over a simple enema is that a greater volume of water flows into the colon. Waste matter and water then run back out past the tubing whenever there is a need to evacuate. The colema board may be purchased from several Internet sites.

Just do a search on "colema" or "colema board."

Colonic Irrigation

Cayce referred to this procedure as a scientific, professional colonic and the most thorough and effective method of cleaning the whole length of the colon. A 61–year–old man (3570) was told that "one colonic irrigation will be worth about four to six enemas."

WHAT A COLONIC DOES

There are several machines on the market that either have a gravity or pressure fill and a siphon/suction return.

Some models use oxygen, which bubbles into the water and kills any pathogenic, anaerobic bacteria. The recommended methods of sanitation are 1) disposable, plastic hoses; 2) sterilizing the rubber hose and metal nozzle in a steam autoclave; and 3) chemical disinfection of the machine after each use. There is no chance of viral or bacterial contamination under these conditions.

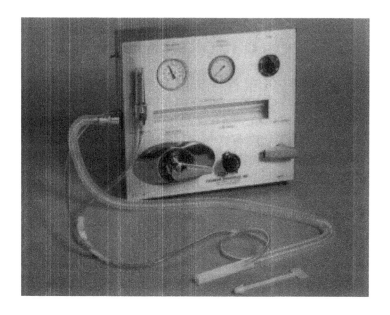

The colon is alternately filled and emptied with water to stretch the pockets and remove any accumulation of mucus and debris. At the same time, the colon muscles are exercised, which, in turn, stimulates peristalsis. This enables the blood and lymph to purify so that the cells can release their waste into a cleaner lymph.

Robert Gray, in his book, *The Colon Health Handbook,* says that whenever there is water in the colon—no matter how much or how little solid matter is removed—a healing reflex action occurs in many parts of the body. This may be due to the many reflex points that are being reached and cleansed during the process. I have found that the eyes and face are particularly responsive to this "enema effect," as Gray calls it. The iris and cornea sparkle and appear brighter, and facial skin often turns a healthy pink. The results are even more dramatic when someone is so toxic that their skin was gray before the session. Occasionally a client will be relieved of a toxic headache (not migraine), or a chronic post-nasal drip will go away, and a person will no longer have the need to clear their throat. Sometimes toxic symptoms will completely clear up during a single session. However, it usually takes a series of colonics to eradicate the problem, as was the case with my bursitis. The possibilities for healing are truly limitless.

One very sensitive client of mine in his mid-thirties has an unusual experience every time he has a colonic. After about ten minutes, he says his aura expands. Then, later on, his chakras open. I feel this happens to everyone when the colon is cleansed, only most of us are not as aware and sensitive as this man is.

In reading 1800-4 Cayce says the human body is made up of electronic vibrations. Whenever there is injury, disease, or *poor eliminations*, then the vibrational energy becomes deficient. This affects the circulation, and inflammation takes place. Thus it only makes sense that whenever toxins are removed, the energy field responds. Almost everyone expresses how much lighter and cleaner they feel afterwards, and this goes far beyond the effect of simply having the physical colon cleansed.

INDICATIONS/CONTRAINDICATIONS

Colonics are particularly helpful during fasting and for the following conditions:

Constipation
Diarrhea (mild)
A sluggish, atonic colon
Mild to moderate hemorrhoids
Intestinal toxemia
Postpartum recovery
Spastic colon
Systemic toxicity.

Colonics are also part of a holistic health approach for many problems such as:

Migraine headaches
Sciatica
Allergies
Sinusitis
Psoriasis
Arthritis.

The A.R.E. Library has a collection of circulating files/research bulletins compiled by physicians on these topics and a variety of other physical ailments.

Colonics may be taken with the approval of a physician or a health care professional for:

Acute fecal impaction
Mucous colitis
Parasitic infestation
Diverticulosis
Ulcerative colitis
Crohn's disease
During the first four months of pregnancy.

ANY ABDOMINAL PAIN SHOULD FIRST BE CHECKED OUT BY A PHYSICIAN.

Colonics are contraindicated for any of the following conditions:

Gastrointestinal bleeding
Cancer of the colon or rectum
Anal fissure or fistula
Abdominal hernia
Acute hemorrhoids
Cardiac disease
Renal insufficiency
Pregnancy after four months
Up to six months after colon or rectal surgery.

ADDITIVES

To purify the system, Cayce insisted that intestinal antiseptics always be added to the water for both enemas and colonics. The additives are poured into the tank of any gravity filling machine. The newer machines have a closed system with a plastic "Y" connector in the clean water line so that any solution may easily be added with a 140 cc syringe or an additive can.

Dissolve well 1 heaping teaspoon salt and 1 level teaspoon baking soda in 1 cup water. Add this to each two quarts of water until the halfway point of the transverse colon is reached.

After the salt/baking soda has been expelled, add 1 tablespoon Glyco-Thymoline to *each* quart of water until the ascending colon is reached.

Lavoris, another alkaline antiseptic, is mentioned nine times in the Cayce readings, but Glyco-Thymoline is recommended 136 times. Alkaline Petrolagar—a combination of mineral oil (petrol) and seaweed (agar)—is recommended 21 times to increase the flow of lymph and to soothe dry and irritated mucous membranes. Two tablespoons are added to the last quart of water either instead of or after the Glyco-Thymoline.

What the combination of salt and baking soda does

Purifies and heals the lymph flow
Reduces the tendency for acidity
Prevents irritation
Strengthens the colon
Prevents too great a reaction of pressure on the hepatic circulation

What Glyco-Thymoline does

Produces a normal lymph circulation
Prevents irritation to the walls after gas pressures are removed
Replenishes and rebuilds the colon walls
Reduces acidity, toxicity, and fermentation
Prevents a strain on the body
Stimulates peristalsis

Cleanses and purifies
Loosens and dissolves mucus

These are extremely important reasons for using the additives, which are not only preventative, but also restore an imbalanced lymph circulation.

A SUMMARY OF CAYCE'S PRECAUTIONS

1) Always add intestinal antiseptics (salt/baking soda and Glyco-Thymoline) to the water to prevent a strain on the body, unless salt is contraindicated for any heart, kidney, or high blood pressure problems.

2) Use body–temperature water.

3) Do not try to clean the whole colon at one time if there are any heart problems.

4) Once the initial series is complete, do not have colonics too often, for dependency may destroy peristalsis. ("Too often" means daily or weekly, for Cayce often advised monthly colonics.)

PREPARATION FOR A COLONIC

Eat lightly for two days before your colonic, and avoid any rich, heavy, or gas–producing food and flour products. The cleansing of the pockets is more effective when there is less matter in the colon.

An enema helps clear the lower colon if there has not been an elimination for several days. It is not necessary to take a laxative, for it has been my experience that laxatives do not always work, and may be more disturbing than helpful.

Abdominal castor oil packs, applied three days in a row before a colonic, will help loosen pocket matter, move lymph, and reduce inflammation. Castor oil was given the name *Palma Christi* or *Palm of Christ* in the Middle Ages because of its healing potential. William McGarey, M.D., author of *Edgar Cayce and the Palma Christi*, was a long-time and well-known advocate of the use of castor oil packs. In his book, *The Oil That Heals*, he asks us to ponder "What kind of healing vibration is there in castor oil that would inspire someone to call the plant the *palm of the Christ*, the Palma Christi?" He goes on to relate a personal story about his young son David, now a physician, who fell down the stairs one night just before bedtime and injured his back. Since there were no neurological symptoms and an x-ray could wait until morning, a castor oil pack was applied. The next morning David was completely fine and totally free of pain. He related that Jesus had come to him in a dream, put His hand on his back, and taken away the pain. Not everyone who uses the packs has a visual healing experience with the Master, but the results continue to be just as miraculous.

ABDOMINAL CASTOR OIL PACK INSTRUCTIONS

Equipment needed:

- 3-4 layers of unbleached, undyed, wool flannel, approximately 12" wide by 14" long. (Use cotton flannel if allergic to wool.) Purchase enough cloth (two packages) to cover from the ribs to the groin and across the expanse of the abdomen. It is preferable for each individual to have his or her own pack.

- 16 oz. of cold-pressed castor oil

- Electric heating pad or a hot water bottle

- Large sheet of plastic (an old shower curtain or a 30-gallon garbage bag)

- Smaller piece of plastic (an old shower curtain or a 30-gallon garbage bag)

- Smaller piece of plastic a couple of inches larger than the cloth, to protect the heating pad from getting oily

- Two bath towels

What to Do

1) Wash and dry the flannel to remove any impurities.

2) Turn on heating pad to the lowest setting.

3) Place smaller plastic on heating pad (or hot water bottle).

4) Place one layer of flannel on plastic. Slowly pour castor oil onto first layer of flannel. Repeat this for each layer so that the pack is thoroughly saturated and the oil is evenly distributed throughout. Each time the pack is used, simply replenish the top layer with oil. Cayce often said to wear rubber gloves, dip the flannel in hot oil and wring it out.

5) Spread the large plastic sheet on the bed and cover with towel.

6) Lie down. Pick up the pile (consisting of flannel, plastic, and heating pad) and place on abdomen with warmed flannel next to skin. If the pack is being used for the liver as well as the colon, make sure the cloth covers the right side of the abdomen.

7) Cover with towel.

8) Leave on 1 to 1½ hours.

9) One's mental attitude is very important. Meditating, praying, reading spiritual material, and a feeling of gratitude are as important as the pack itself. Cayce also wanted us to learn how the body functions so that we can see it working in the way that is desired. Today this is called "visualization" and its value in healing and in improving physical performance (honing basketball skills, for example) is well-documented. Positive expectations are vital. He encouraged one to *expect* to be healed and not to be discouraged by any physical symptoms. Ruth O'Lill's wonderful book, *A Personal Guide to Hope: Where to Find It , How to Keep It*, offers specific examples of this in her "Hope is Healing" chapter. Her book shows us eighteen different ways that hope can steer us safely through the troubled waters of life and into a calm, more serene place.

10) After removing the pack, wash the skin with a solution of 1

teaspoon baking soda dissolved in 1 cup warm water to prevent any skin reactions.

11) Take 2 teaspoons olive oil at bedtime.

12) After 3 days' use, store the flannel in a glass jar. You may also refrigerate it, if desired.

THE COLONIC SESSION

Since a full stomach may cause discomfort during a colonic, it is advisable not to eat for two hours ahead of time. The appointment usually lasts an hour.

A long, hospital–type gown is worn, with an optional covering over the legs.

As you lie on your left side, a 2–inch, lubricated nozzle is inserted into the rectum.

There are two hoses: a clean water line and a waste line. A gauge monitors the water as it gradually fills and empties the colon. The water can be released any time there is a feeling of fullness. As waste matter is removed, there is more room for the next fill. The colon can hold 1½ to 2½ quarts of water.

You may either remain on your left side, or turn on your back so that the colon can be massaged to help release gas and water.

On those occasions when . . .

Once in a long while, the water does not release quickly and easily because a gas pocket or bubble holds it back. If this happens, one or more of the following suggestions may be helpful for you and your therapist.

For You:

1) Take several long, deep, relaxing breaths through the nose.

2) Gently press and hold your colon hand reflex points with your opposite thumb for 10-60 seconds. The point on the back of the left hand is pressed first, to relax the descending colon and half of the

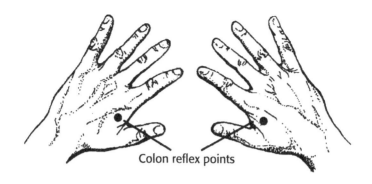

Colon reflex points

transverse colon. Then the point on the right hand is pressed to relax the other half of the transverse, along with the ascending colon.

For Your Therapist:

1) Gently pull up under the splenic flexure, and hold the stretch for 5-10 seconds. This move allows the splenic flexure to reposition so that the transverse colon can release more easily.

2) Apply 2 drops of Bach Flower Rescue Remedy, a homeopathic flower essence, on the inside of the client's wrist, then have him/her touch both wrists together for 1 to 2 seconds. Several drops may also be placed at 2- to 3-inch intervals along the colon area of the abdomen.

3) Alternately press the colon foot reflex points (page 98) from the cecum to the rectum with your thumb 2 to 3 times.

4) Slowly circle a chlorite crystal over the colon area, starting at the cecum. The chlorite is a clear quartz crystal with deposits of green chlorophyll that enhance healing. The chlorite acts as a laser when the point is directed towards a specific area, or it can draw out negativity when the flat, base-cut end is placed on an area of imbalance. The chlorite is unique, for it continues to send healing energy to an area long after a session is complete. Before and after each use, it should be cleansed by placing it in a bowl of salt for 24 hours, or by running pure water over it. It should not be placed in sunlight.

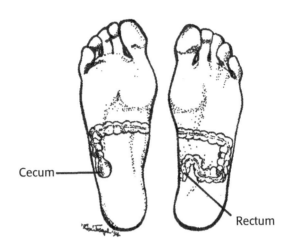

Cecum

Rectum

5) Stop to allow the client to use the bathroom. This can be very effective in relieving gas.

Flower and Gemstone Essences

Flower essences are made from individual plant flowers that are placed in pure water in direct sunlight for three to four hours. Their specific healing pattern is released vibrationally into the water. This "tincture" is then diluted, preserved in brandy or vinegar, and taken orally, a few drops at a time. Flower essences work on the mental and emotional levels to release patterns that cause illness on the physical level. They also help to reconnect weakened, electrical nerve impulses, and rebalance any overload of electrical impulses along the spine.

Gemstone essences are made from specific gemstones that are placed in pure water in direct sunlight for one to two hours. Their essence is imparted vibrationally into the water in the same manner as the flowers. The following are especially helpful for the colon:

- Smoky quartz   Clears negativity
- Amethyst   Protects from and clears negativity
- Clear quartz   Imparts solidified LIGHT
- Rose quartz   Imparts universal LOVE

Kinesiology (muscle testing that is thoroughly explained in Machaelle Small Wright's book, *Flower Essences*) is one method that can be used to determine which flower and gemstone essences are needed.

AFTER THE COLONIC

One can anticipate feeling more peaceful, lighter, cleaner, and more energized after a colonic. On rare occasions, if there has been a longstanding condition of constipation or several health problems, a slight headache or some fatigue may be experienced with the first or second colonic. If this is so, a short rest will help restore one's equilibrium.

Since the colon has been cleared of solid matter, it may take one or two days before it fills up again and normal bowel movements are resumed. Some water is absorbed through the colon wall during a colonic, and one may notice an increased need to urinate for a few hours afterwards. This beneficial effect of flushing the kidneys may also be enhanced by drinking a few glasses of water with the juice of half a lemon added to each glass.

A colonic has a profound cleansing effect on the body, and many people feel so good afterwards that they want to double their jogging or work-out time. Caution is advised here, for it can be overdone. Although light to moderate exercise is good if you are used to it, any strenuous activity should be avoided that day.

A light diet of fruits, vegetables, salads, soup, and chicken or fish should be followed for two days, taking care to avoid anything that causes gas. Rich or heavy food, flour products, spices, and alcohol should also be omitted. Although irrigating the colon does not remove all of the intestinal bacteria, it is still often helpful to take some form of acidophilus to maintain bacterial balance. In addition, Cayce advised yogurt because it is an active cleanser that also adds vital forces to the colon.

How often one should have a colonic depends on the diet, stress level, health, age, and how successful the colonic was. Cayce often advised having colonics until mucus is no longer visible in the release water. He generally recommended an initial series of three to six, or sometimes eight—one every seven to ten days, before going on a maintenance program. A maintenance colonic can be done once or twice a year, at the change of seasons, or monthly. Most people seem to know when they need to come again.

One of my clients shared her feelings about what colonics are like for her:

> The first experience seemed uneventful, though the colonic machine confronted a body staunchly defending years of the accumulative effects of a faulty diet, stress, and an overload of drugs from various health challenges I had struggled to overcome. Having now been introduced to the benefit of castor oil packs as a preparation for a colonic, including vegetables and whole grains as the mainstay of my diet, and begun walking for exercise, the results of the second session, two weeks later, were dramatic. I not only permanently decreased a size in clothing, but for the first time my skin was now clear, my eyes shone, and there was a vitality I vaguely remembered having only as a child.
>
> Twelve years have passed since opening up to health as a possibility. It is now a way of life I choose to pursue. I realize it pursues me, as well, for whenever I veer off into old habit patterns, I am beset by the same warning signals as before: lethargy, bloating, melancholy, restlessness, discontent, skin eruptions, etc. The contrast I feel when released from this sluggish build-up is not as dramatic as my first encounter with colon therapy, but the assured outcome of each treatment is always a restorative balance of calm and well-being.

Summary

1) A 2-quart enema is the simplest method of irrigating the colon.

2) Other types of enemas are coffee, medicated, oil retention, and three-stage.

3) A colon tube, or high enema, cleanses the colon and stimulates peristalsis more effectively than a low enema.

4) A colema uses a greater volume of water than a simple enema.

5) A colonic, worth four to six enemas, is the most thorough and effective method of cleansing the colon.

6) Colonics expand and cleanse the colon pockets, tone up colon muscles, stimulate peristalsis, and purify the blood and lymph.

7) There are several precautions and contraindications to be noted.

8) Salt/baking soda and Glyco-Thymoline should be added to the enema/colonic (unless salt is contraindicated).

9) Colonics are more effective with castor oil packs as a preparation.

10) A colonic is an energizing experience, as one's body is freed from the effects of its own toxicity.

11) Deep breathing, hand and foot reflexology on the colon areas, and other aids help the colon relax and release.

NINE

Constipation

. . . for [if] the assimilations and the eliminations would be kept nearer normal in the human family, the days might be extended to whatever period as was so desired; for the system is builded by the assimilations of that it takes within, and is able to bring resuscitations so long as the eliminations do not hinder.

311-4

More people come for a colonic because of infrequent and difficult eliminations than for any other reason. Constipation is a very troublesome condition, causing hemorrhoids, diverticulosis, diverticulitis, impaction, toxemia, and prolapsus. Even more important, poor eliminations are at the root of most diseases.

If sluggish eliminations continue over a period of time, the rectum becomes distended and the urge to evacuate diminishes. A progressively worsening domino effect now occurs: the colon tends to narrow or balloon out as matter backs up, the transverse section sags, the ascending colon enlarges, and the colon becomes distorted into many different shapes.

A BADLY CONSTIPATED COLON

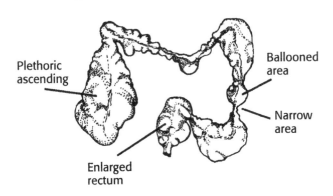

Causes of Constipation

There are several factors contributing to constipation. Although not all conditions will be present in each individual's case, a common pattern from the readings emerges:

1) Poor diet
2) Dryness of the colon lymph due to acidity
3) Excess toxins
4) Torpid liver with decreased bile production
5) Insufficient water intake
6) Lack of exercise
7) Nervous tension and stress
8) Spinal misalignment
9) Negative attitudes and emotions

The first four conditions:

1) Poor diet
2) Dryness of the colon lymph due to acidity
3) Excess toxins
4) Torpid liver with decreased bile production

are closely interwoven, for a diet low in fiber and high in starch, fat,

CAUSES OF CONSTIPATION

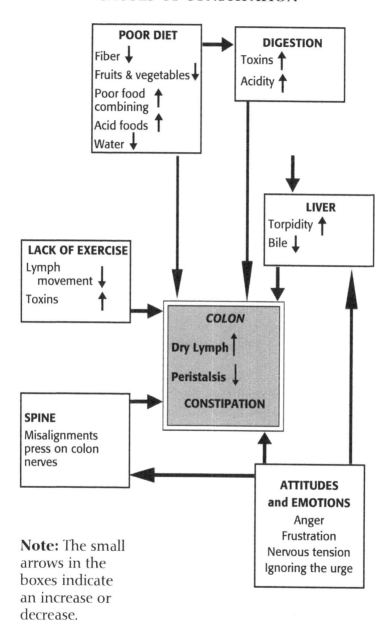

Note: The small arrows in the boxes indicate an increase or decrease.

and meat creates a highly acidic condition. This dries out the lymph in the colon, peristalsis slows down, and toxicity develops. Many of the toxins in the colon are now reabsorbed into the blood, which overwhelms the liver. It cannot then adequately produce bile, which is nature's laxative.

An insufficient intake of water (condition #5) causes the stool to become dry and hard. Many times a temporary sluggishness can be alleviated by just drinking more water.

A lack of exercise (condition #6) decreases the colon's muscle tone and slows down the movement of lymph fluid.

And the last three conditions:

7) Nervous tension and stress
8) Spinal misalignment
9) Negative attitudes and emotions

are also closely connected, for stress, tension, and negative emotions contract both colon and back muscles. The resulting spinal misalignments put pressure on nerves that affect the colon, slowing down peristalsis. Cayce often recommended osteopathic adjustments because they will redistribute energy so that more normal eliminations can occur.

Let me share a client's story of how the emotional stress of a financial situation literally shut down her colon. "Marlene" had sold her house for a generous profit, but was unable to find a secure investment that would allow her to live off of the income. Still, for three months, she felt very secure, until one day she decided to sit down and add up some figures. Much to her surprise, the data revealed that she had already spent over 25 percent of her capital, which lowered the amount of her monthly income. The shock of this discovery manifested immediately in her colon, and she became constipated for several days.

She decided to meditate and ask why her colon was in trouble. As she mentally envisioned this area, she noticed that it was blue instead of a normal, healthy pink. The colon communicated that it was cold and frightened because of the shock and money fears she had dumped there. This insight enabled her to let go of all these negative emotions.

The emotional release allowed her colon to relax, and she was able to have a bowel movement shortly thereafter.

What to Do for Constipation

DIET

- Drink 1–2 glasses orange juice daily
- Drink 1–2 oz. carrot juice daily
- Drink 4–8 glasses of water daily
- Eat raw fruits and vegetables
- Increase fiber intake
- Properly combine food (see Chapter 5)
- Do not use spices, which dry out the lymph
- Take olive oil in small doses of ¼ to ½ teaspoon every 2–3 hours for 3 days to stimulate the release of bile.

COLON

Since it has taken a while for constipation to develop, it will require a commitment of time and energy to reverse this condition. Have an initial series of 6 to 8 colonics, 7 to 10 days apart, to restore peristalsis, remove toxins, cleanse the liver, and improve digestion. The schedule of maintenance colonics varies with the individual.

Use castor oil packs three days in a row before each colonic to stimulate the lymph flow in the colon.

SPINE

Have osteopathic adjustments once or twice a week to these areas of the spine: C3, T4 through T12, L1 and L2. It may be difficult to find an osteopath in your area, but Cayce preferred this method of spinal manipulation. However, there may be a chiropractor in your area who is familiar with this treatment. (See under "Resources" in the Appendix for obtaining the A.R.E.'s list of cooperating health care professionals.)

EXERCISE

Take daily morning walks in the open air, swim, go biking, golfing, or rowing.

Yoga abdominal lifts are very beneficial for strengthening the abdominal and colon muscles. They must be done before a meal, when the stomach is empty.

To do the abdominal lifts:
- Bend over and place hands on mid thighs.
- Exhale as completely as you can.
- While holding the exhalation, pump the abdomen in and out several times.
- Relax and breathe normally.
- Repeat two or three times.

ATTITUDES AND EMOTIONS

Pay attention to the urge to evacuate—don't ignore it or wait for a more convenient time.

Positive emotions will keep the liver happy, the colon relaxed, and the spine aligned.

Have a daily period of quiet time, contemplation, and meditation. The benefits are far-reaching. One may discover that he or she is holding on to a job, money, or a relationship because of a lack of trust. This feeling causes the colon to hold on as well. When there is a "letting go" of fear and worry on the mental/emotional level, the colon responds in kind.

A 61-year-old man (3570) asked a very interesting question of Cayce:

> Is there any organic irregularity, dislocation, adhesion, or other complication of the digestive or intestinal tract which is and has been causing almost nonexistent natural elimination for years?

He suspected that all of his complaints were connected to his elimination problems, and there were many. He suffered from frequent, severe headaches; shortness of breath; rapid heartbeat; gastric upset; eczema on his right elbow, and soreness in the back of his neck.

Cayce's reply was that he was "in part starving to death." Since any grain seemed to further aggravate his symptoms, he had already eliminated grains from his diet and ate mostly soybean flour, fruits, vegetables, milk, meat, and fish—which sounds like a fairly good diet. But Cayce informed him that he was not absorbing the nutrients from his food, and this was causing a form of starvation.

The man related that his physical problems had started years before when he overloaded his body with acids by eating too much meat, grease, and starches, and stomach ulcers formed.

Ironically, eating mostly fruits and vegetables made matters worse because these foods fermented in his stomach and small intestine, irritating the ulcers. This improper digestion smoothed out the walls of the duodenum and inhibited peristalsis. It is not surprising that the man had terrible headaches, pressure in his neck, and heart problems!

The treatment, however, was quite simple:

1) Frequent, small doses of olive oil (½ teaspoon, 4-6 times a day) to heal the mucous membranes and balance the flow of lymph through the alimentary canal
2) Castor oil packs over the liver and gall duct area
3) Beef juice (see method of preparation in Chapter 11)
4) Chicken broth
5) Colonic irrigations to remove reflex pressures on the heart and prostate gland.

Cayce told Mr. 3570 that although his health could be 40 percent better, his improvement shouldn't be limited to his physical health. Instead, he was advised to be not just good, but "good for something," and practice what he preached for the benefit of everyone, not just a few friends that thought like *he* did. Often when a person came to Cayce seeking a "cure," Cayce would turn the focus around, ask the seeker why he or she wanted to get better, and just what changes in the life would be made if the person *were* healed. It's a thought-provoking question.

Hemorrhoids

Hemorrhoids are dilated veins that occur externally or internally in the anus and rectum. They result from straining during constipation, and commonly occur during pregnancy. They may periodically cause pain, itching, and bleeding.

Cayce attributed hemorrhoids not only to constipation, but also to hyperacidity, anxiety, nervousness, stress, and a disturbance between the liver and kidneys. Surgery was advised in only two out of 65 cases, which is encouraging. The others were told that if the guidance were followed, they would either be cured or there would be a more normal condition.

WHAT TO DO FOR HEMORRHOIDS
Tim Ointment

Tim Ointment contains iodine, tincture of benzoin, tobacco, and butterfat, which help shrink the swollen tissue, alleviate pain, and restore normal conditions. It may be applied daily or after each bowel movement. After each application, one should lie down with the feet elevated to a level above the head. "Consistently used, it will not only remove the cause but remove the hemorrhoids," affirms reading 257-200 for a 45-year-old male.

A 34-year-old woman, in reading 457-9, was given the following formula to cure her hemorrhoids. It may be used as an ointment and occasionally injected into the rectum.

To 1 oz. of glycerine, add 2 drops of carbolic acid. Stir well.

Add 1 oz. of Russian White Oil (mineral oil). Stir.

Exercise

Do the following exercise very slowly 3 times in the morning and 3 times in the evening. This gradually lifts the sphincter muscles and heals the hemorrhoids.

- Inhale as you rise on tiptoe and raise arms overhead.

- Still on tiptoe, exhale as you bend over and touch your toes. Bend only as far as comfortable.

- Still on tiptoe, inhale as you come back up and raise arms overhead.

- Exhale as you bring arms to sides and lower the heels to the floor.

Sitz Baths (See "Prostatitis" in Chapter 7.)

Colonics

Have a series of 3 to 6 colonics, 7 to 10 days apart.

Spine

Have osteopathic adjustments to the lumbar, sacrum, and coccyx.

Castor Oil Packs

Cut a small piece of flannel from your castor oil pack and tuck it snugly against the hemorrhoid. Wear a sanitary pad to safeguard clothing, and change the flannel daily.

Gas/Flatulence

Taber's Cyclopedic Medical Dictionary defines flatulence as gas in the digestive tract due to fermentation or decomposition. Most people have some degree of gas, even severe gas, at times.

Cayce, who was asked approximately 150 times what could be done for this problem, primarily attributed the presence of gas to a lack of hydrochloric acid and gastric juices in the stomach and small intestine, preventing proper digestion. As the food then ferments, bacteria and gas multiply and disturb the acid/alkaline balance.

Even if there is an adequate supply of stomach acid and gastric juices, when food is eaten in improper combination with other foods (see Chapter 5), it does not digest properly and forms gas. For this reason, Cayce advised not eating more than one starch at a meal, and often warned against large quantities of starch, especially bread, for it clogs the system and causes a lack of reaction in the colon, resulting in gas.

Although raw food is good for us, it may cause gas in an already congested colon. Many foods naturally produce more gas than others, especially when uncooked, but this does not mean we should avoid eating these nutritious foods.

GAS-PRODUCING FOODS

Raw apples	Cauliflower
Bananas	Cucumbers
Beans, dried	Melons
Broccoli	Onions
Brussels sprouts	Peppers
Cabbage	Unripened fruit

We also need to consider the effects of our emotions on the digestive process. Even foods that digest well when we are relaxed will potentially cause gas when we are worried or in a fearful state.

WHAT TO DO FOR GAS

Diet

- Combine food properly (See Chapter 5).
- Drink liquids between meals, not with meals, so that the gastric juices will not be diluted.
- Eat when relaxed, and have a quiet time afterwards.
- Chew food thoroughly to enhance the production of an adequate amount of digestive juices.
- Orange juice, with 1 to 2 tablespoons lemon juice per glass, will keep down the tendency for gas to form in the alimentary canal.

Colonics

A regular maintenance schedule of colonics will not only keep down the tendency for gas to accumulate, but will remove mucus, which causes gas.

Charcoal

Activated charcoal capsules, tablets, or powder may help absorb gas, but should be considered only as a short–term remedy—limited to 3 months if taken on a daily basis. Capsules are almost twice as potent as the tablets.

Castor Oil Pack

A castor oil pack, worn overnight without heat, may offer relief in an acute situation.

Cold Abdominal Compress

The following procedure may be helpful in an acute episode:

Soak a small towel in a bowl of ice water, wring out, and apply to the abdomen.
Wrap a large, Turkish towel around the body and leave on overnight. Repeat as needed.

Diverticulosis

Diverticulosis is a condition in which pea–sized sacs called *diverticula* develop in the wall of the lower descending colon and sigmoid colon. They occur when the colon has to strain in order to push hard, constipated stool along. This eventually weakens the muscles, and diverticula herniate in the wall of the colon.

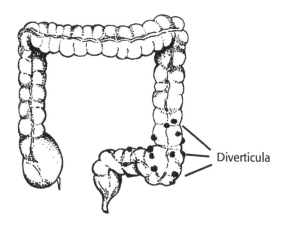

Diverticula

Diverticulitis

Diverticulitis results when fecal matter becomes trapped and stagnates in the diverticula. An acute episode occurs when there is inflammation, abdominal pain, infection, and fever. It can be treated medically with a low fiber or liquid diet, antibiotics, bed rest, or hospitalization. Castor oil packs for 3–4 hours at a time for 3–4 days may also be helpful.

WHAT TO DO FOR DIVERTICULOSIS AND DIVERTICULITIS
Diet
- Eat fruits and vegetables, high fiber foods, and whole grains.
- Avoid processed food, white flour products, and junk food.
- Avoid popcorn, seeds, and nuts that can collect in the diverticula.

Castor Oil Packs
Apply castor oil packs for 1½ hours three days in a row as needed for a maintenance routine.

Colonics
After a 3-day series of castor oil packs—and only upon a physician's referral—have *gentle* colonics once or twice a week for 2 to 3 weeks, then once a month for 2 to 3 months.

Spine
Have osteopathic manipulations once or twice a week for 3 to 4 weeks, rest 2 weeks, and repeat. This series is to be repeated 3 to 4 times.

Massage
Have a full-body massage—with emphasis on Cayce's spinal massage (gentle circle friction from C1 to L5)—using equal parts peanut oil and olive oil, once or twice a week, for 5 to 6 weeks. Repeat as necessary.

Prolapsus

A prolapsus is a dropping or sagging of any section of the colon; however, it happens more frequently in the transverse colon because of the heavy weight of constipated stool. The two bends in the colon then have a sharper angle that impedes the smooth passage of stool. Prolapsus may also be caused by nervous indigestion, fear, iron deficiency, and spinal misalignments at T6, T7, and T8. A heavy feeling may be experienced in the abdomen and back if the prolapsed area presses on the bladder, uterus, or prostate gland.

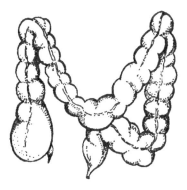

WHAT TO DO FOR A PROLAPSUS

Colonics

Colonics are given gradually and slowly so that 2 to 3 are required to reach the whole colon. The frequency is once a week for 4 to 6 weeks, followed by a maintenance schedule of once a month for 3 to 4 months.

Exercise

Do yoga abdominal lifts (see page 108) 1 or 2 times a day. They are particularly helpful.

Slant Board

Another approach to rectifying a prolapsed colon is to use a slant board. Exercises are done lying down, which allows the transverse colon and abdominal organs to fall back into their proper position.

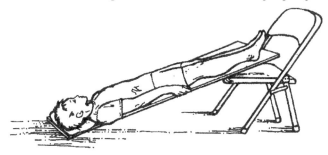

One lies with the head at the lower end and the feet elevated, which will also increase circulation to the brain.

A board should not be used if there is heart disease, high blood pressure, hemorrhage, history of stroke, tuberculosis, pregnancy, herniation, pelvic cancer, or any condition in which blood to the head would be contraindicated.

Commercial models may be purchased, or a supportive flat board may be used by elevating one end to chair height. It should have an adequate length and width to comfortably accommodate the body.

Begin slowly by just lying on the slant board once a day for one minute. If a headache or dizziness is experienced at first, do not raise the feet as high. Then, over several weeks, gradually increase the time to 10 minutes, twice a day.

After you feel comfortable, "bicycling" with the legs or bending the knees up and down may be slowly introduced. Repeat 5 to 10 times while holding onto the side of the board.

The colon may also be massaged 3 to 4 times. Stroke and pull up on the ascending colon with the fingertips, push across the transverse colon with the heel of the right hand, then push down on the descending colon with the heel of the left hand.

Summary

1) Constipation is a troublesome condition that, in turn, causes other health problems.

2) An acidic diet and poor digestion cause a dryness of the colon lymph, which is the main cause of constipation.

3) The liver then becomes torpid and produces insufficient bile, which is nature's laxative.

4) Lack of exercise, insufficient water intake, spinal misalignment, and negative attitudes and emotions all play their part in constipation.

5) Hemorrhoids, or dilated veins in the anus and rectum, are caused by constipation, hyperacidity, stress, and a disturbance between the liver and kidneys. Tim Ointment and specific exercises are helpful.

6) Flatulence, or gas, is caused by a lack of stomach acid and gastric juices, and by improper food combining.

7) Proper diet and colonics help alleviate the cause of gas. Castor oil packs without heat, or a cold abdominal compress, may be helpful in acute situations.

8) Diverticulosis develops when the colon strains in order to push hard, constipated stool along. Fecal matter becomes trapped and stagnates in the diverticula.

9) Diverticulosis can be prevented by a diet high in fiber, fruits, and vegetables.

10) Diverticulitis results when trapped fecal matter in the diverticula causes inflammation, abdominal pain, infection, and fever.

11) A prolapsus occurs when the transverse colon sags from the weight of heavy, constipated stool. Gentle, gradual colonics and slant board exercises are beneficial.

TEN

Laxatives

For those conditions that have become rather as habits, and those tendencies or necessities for the body to use the eliminants—or those things that tend to make for the flow of the gastric forces or the peristaltic movement through the intestinal system (for we find that much of this is habit, and the body, the system has come to depend upon cathartics), we would create for the system that which will cooperate in making for better coordination with the adjustments and treatments as indicated . . .

Then make for self a regular period, after the morning meal, for the evacuation or for going to stool, see? Let this be as a habit. Let this be taking the place of the cathartics and the like.

777-3

Cayce's Viewpoint

The need to take something in order to have a bowel movement has created a laxative industry with sales of eight billion dollars a year. Constipation was a problem in Cayce's day, as well, for he discussed the pros and cons of laxatives in almost 2900 readings.

He felt that any eliminant merely stimulates the activity of the mucous membranes to produce more lymph, which takes the vitality out of the very system it is necessary to strengthen, namely the lymphatics. When the lymph has been overexcited, peristalsis declines even further, and eventually a soreness is created in the colon.

What seems to help at first only contributes to a long-term problem. Laxatives lose their effectiveness when used regularly, requiring larger and larger doses to produce the same result. Eventually, this dependency inhibits the natural functioning of the colon. At this point, many people turn to harsher cathartics, such as Epsom salts or castor oil—which Cayce warned against using—for they not only irritate the muscles, but congest the circulation between the liver and kidneys.

Laxative Foods

When asked what laxative was best to take, he often responded that "the best laxative is a balanced diet" (457-9) and, beyond that, to eat more foods that have a laxative effect, such as

Figs, stewed or raw
Prunes
Raisins
Rhubarb stems
Sauerkraut juice
Leafy, green vegetables (kale, collards, beet tops, parsley, watercress, spinach, turnip greens, dandelion greens, Swiss chard, mustard greens, wild greens, endive, escarole, etc.)
Fresh citrus juice
Fresh carrot juice
Mummy food (See explanation on next page.)

These foods are most effective when rotated. For example, on Monday and Tuesday, have stewed prunes or warm prune juice; Wednesday and Thursday, drink two to three glasses of orange or grapefruit juice. (Remember to not drink citrus juice at the same meal with cereal or milk.) Friday, Saturday, and Sunday, have freshly squeezed carrot juice. The following week, vary leafy green vegetables with mummy food or stewed rhubarb, etc.

Fruits are the cleansers and have a laxative effect; vegetables are the builders, containing more minerals than fruits do.

JUICES

A 66-year-old woman (5592) was told that citrus, taken in its season, is nature's laxative, and that a cathartic would not be necessary if at least one meal a day consisted only of citrus.

One to two ounces of fresh, raw carrot juice a day was advised several times in the readings to stimulate better eliminations and dissolve poisons and toxins. In partial contrast with Cayce, Dr. Norman Walker, D.Sc.—a pioneer in the health field in his book, *Fresh Vegetable and Fruit Juices*, says that large amounts of carrot juice aids digestion and helps in the treatment of intestinal and liver disorders, ulcers, and cancer. He feels that the best food for the colon is a combination of 10 ounces of carrot juice and 6 ounces of spinach juice. Depending on one's health, one to eight pints are taken daily, in addition to salads and vegetables.

Spinach juice effectively cleanses and helps heal the whole intestinal tract. Carrot juice is a major detoxifier of the liver and dissolver of toxins. Dr. Walker recommends that all fresh juice be consumed shortly after being squeezed, to prevent fermentation and loss of nutrients.

MUMMY FOOD

The following recipe was given to Cayce in a dream in which a female mummy came to life and gave instructions for making a food she required—a food basic to the Atlanteans and ancient Egyptians, according to the readings.

Mummy Food Recipe, from Reading 1907-2

Mix together in a saucepan:
   1 cup chopped, black Syrian figs
   1 cup chopped dates (Do not use pitted dates; remove pits just before chopping)
Add: ½ cup water and bring almost to a boil
Add: 1 rounded tablespoon yellow cornmeal and stir well
Cook 10–15 minutes, stirring frequently.

Cayce thought so highly of mummy food that he referred to it as almost a spiritual food. It stimulates the eliminations, purifies the system of refuse or ash forces, and prevents gas from forming. A small quantity eaten as a cereal with milk or cream was specifically given to help build strength in children and elderly individuals.

Constipating Foods

Certain foods are more constipating than others and should be eaten in moderation or avoided altogether:

Bananas
Carob
Cheese
Chocolate
Coffee
Fried food
White flour

Pod vegetables (beans, peas, etc.)
Potatoes (the skins by themselves
    are not constipating)
Pickles, spices and condiments
    (which hinder the flow of
    lymph in the colon)

Eliminants

Laxatives were occasionally recommended for a short period of time while other measures, such as diet, colonics, spinal adjustments, and exercise, had a chance to correct the underlying cause of constipation. He felt that gentler laxatives help stimulate a more normal evacuation without cramping or irritation. Four groups of eliminants are mentioned:

Eliminant	Quantity of Readings
Mechanical Laxatives (bulk-forming or lubricant)	671
Vegetable base	900
Mineral base	75
Fruit base	225

One should be aware that long-term use of laxatives may result in becoming dependent on them. Consult your doctor if pregnant or nursing a baby. Avoid laxatives altogether if there is any:

> Abdominal pain
> Nausea
> Vomiting
> Rectal bleeding
> Kidney disease
> Diarrhea or constipation lasting two weeks.

MECHANICAL LAXATIVES

Mechanical laxatives fall into two categories: bulk forming and lubricant. They are the most natural and least irritating to the intestinal tract.

Bulk-forming laxatives absorb water in the intestines and swell to form a soft, bulky stool. This gives a natural feeling of fullness that stimulates the colon to evacuate.

Lubricant laxatives are oils that coat the stool with a waterproof film. This allows the stool to retain moisture and stay soft, enabling it to pass through the colon more easily. Though castor oil coats the stool, it is a harsh cathartic and irritates the small intestine. Olive oil is the laxative of choice in the readings.

Olive Oil (500 readings)

Olive oil is a food for mucous membranes and helps counteract dryness in the colon. A pure oil (the first pressing of organic olives) is taken in small doses of ¼ to ½ teaspoon, four or five times a day, for two to three days, left off for two to three days, then repeated. This maintains the flow of bile, which is itself a laxative, and helps rid the gallbladder of gravel. In reading 644, Cayce says that it would be well for everybody to occasionally take olive oil in this manner.

Mineral Oil (113 readings)

Cayce preferred three brand names of mineral oil that, unfortunately, are no longer available: Nujol, Usoline, and Russian White Oil. He cautioned, however, that the oil should only be used in moderation, so as not to become dependent upon it. Although mineral oil is widely used, it has been found that long-term use prevents absorption of vitamins A, D, E, and K.

Castor Oil (20 readings)

Caution: DO NOT TAKE INTERNALLY WHEN PREGNANT.

Known as the Palma Christi, or Palm of Christ, Cayce generally advised using castor oil externally—as a pack, rather than internally—because it is a harsh cathartic.

Psyllium (38 readings)

Psyllium is a powder made from the crushed seeds of the herb *plantain* that swells when mixed with water or juice to produce bulk and weight. This improves peristalsis without producing too much roughage and dilation of the colon. The husk is more effective than the seed. Cayce preferred blonde psyllium, *plantago ovata*, because it is more palatable.

Current usage is anywhere from 1 teaspoon up to 2 tablespoons of psyllium stirred into a glass of diluted fruit juice and swallowed immediately, before it thickens. It is then followed with a glass of water.

Cayce's directions, however, are to stir 1 tablespoon of powder into 4 tablespoons of hot water or milk, and allow to jell for 5 to 10 minutes. It can then be eaten alone or added to the breakfast cereal. It may be taken twice a day, preferably at breakfast and supper.

If one has severe constipation or a prolapsus, one should not use psyllium until the muscle tone and functioning of the colon have improved.

VEGETABLE BASE

Fletcher's Castoria (300 readings)

Fletcher's Castoria is a mild, children's laxative that Cayce recommended *for adults.* The main ingredient is senna, a non-habit-forming stimulant laxative that increases peristalsis. It is taken in small doses of ½ to 1 teaspoon every 30 or 60 minutes, and it may take 6 to 8 hours before an elimination occurs.

Senna (200 readings)

Cayce indicated that senna does not become habit-forming, as do other laxatives, and is a good choice for most individuals.

Pods: Pour boiling water over 3 to 4 pods; let stand 30–40 minutes, then strain and drink as a tea.

Dried leaves: Either chew them and follow with a glass of water or make into a tea: pour boiling water over a teaspoonful, let sit for 5 minutes, strain and drink.

Senna may also be purchased in capsule form at most health food stores.

Podophyllum (125 readings)

Also known as Mandrake or May Apple, Podophyllum acts upon the liver to increase the flow of bile. Since it irritates the duodenum to increase the intestinal secretions, it is now only available by prescription.

Ragweed (100 readings)

Also called Ambrosia Weed, Ragweed is a non–habit–forming, bitter weed that aids digestion and the entire eliminating system. According to Cayce, it is the best vegetable compound for the liver. A 48–year–old man (644) was told that if it were taken fresh and green as part of the diet or as a medicine, then appendicitis would never occur.

Zilatone (75 readings)

Zilatone is a laxative compound that contains bile extract, cascara sagrada, pancreatin, pepsin, phenolphthalein and capsicum. It stimulates the liver, pancreas, and spleen and corrects the incoordination among the eliminating systems. It also aids digestion if quantities of water are consumed at the same time.

Cascara Sagrada (100 readings)

Found in several formulas in the readings, Cascara Sagrada is a mild, stimulant laxative that acts on the intestinal wall to increase peristalsis. It is available in most health food stores.

MINERAL BASE
Caroid and Bile Salts (100 readings)

Now known as Caroid Laxative, this laxative contains phenolphthalein and cascara sagrada; however the digestive ingredients have been removed from the formula. In Cayce's day, it contained caroid, capsicum, bile salts, phenolphthalein, and cascara sagrada, all of which help to digest protein, stimulate the flow of bile, and clean the whole system.

Sal Hepatica (100 readings)

Sal Hepatica is a saline laxative that draws water into the bowel from the surrounding tissues, creating a rapid emptying of the colon. A 53-year-old woman (1770-6) asked if it were harmful to take every morning. Cayce responded that sauerkraut juice would be just as saline and would stimulate better eliminations.

As a child, Cayce fell on a stick. The healing was slow, and left a clot, adhesions, and a stricture in the intestines. As a result, he suffered for years from poor eliminations and headaches. One of the laxatives his own readings suggested was Sal Hepatica.

Sulflax (75 readings)

This is a mild laxative and blood purifier that contains equal parts of sulfur, cream of tartar, and Rochelle salts. It is frequently indicated for acne, boils, eczema, psoriasis, and dermatitis to stimulate and coordinate the eliminations. Interestingly, Cayce cautioned against getting the feet wet in the rain or swimming while taking it, although bathing was allowed.

FRUIT BASE
Eno Salts (150 readings)

Cayce preferred the fruit salts variety; however, it is no longer available in this country. The formula has been changed and is now simply an antacid.

Syrup of Rhubarb (75 readings)

Rhubarb is highly regarded in herbal books. The dried, powdered root comes from northern China and Tibet. Only small amounts are used, for it can be very irritating.

Summary

1) Laxatives generate sales of eight billion dollars a year. Cayce gave almost 2900 readings on the subject.

2) Laxatives and cathartics stimulate the mucous membranes to produce more lymph. This ultimately contributes to constipation, for peristalsis is slowed down further.

3) When laxatives are used on a daily basis, larger amounts are required, and effectiveness is eventually lost. Cayce did not approve of cathartics, for they are more harsh and irritating.

4) Cayce often recommended laxative-producing foods, such as citrus, carrot juice, mummy food, figs, and green leafy vegetables.

5) Four groups of laxatives are suggested in the readings to be used for short periods of time while corrective measures are being followed.

6) Olive oil, taken in small, frequent doses, is the most frequently recommended laxative in the readings.

ELEVEN

Colitis

In the physical forces of the body—these respond so long as there are the precautionary measures kept in the manner which has been indicated. When there is neglect, overindulgence or the disregarding of the warnings, there are those disturbing conditions in which the inclinations have been indicated that become a part of the experience.   *257-202*

Irritable bowel syndrome, or I.B.S., is a name given by the medical community to cover a whole complex of symptoms that used to be individually labeled mucous colitis, spastic colitis, spastic colon, ulcerative colitis, and non-inflammatory diarrhea.

Colitis, or I.B.S., actually means inflammation of the colon and is accompanied by bouts of diarrhea, constipation, fever, and abdominal discomfort or pain. In an acute attack, there may be as many as 15 to 20 liquid stools a day. Ulcerative colitis is more severe, for the mucous lining thickens, ulcerates, and bleeds, leaving the colon thick and rigid from scar tissue.

Colitis is usually preceded by a cold or intestinal flu, according to Cayce, and there is always a disturbance in the intestinal lymphatics (lymph nodes, lacteal ducts and Peyer's patches) when the inflammation occurs. The lymph then becomes toxic, adversely affecting the liver, and causes nausea, hyperacidity, and poor assimilation. As a result, excess mucus is produced by the colon as a protection against the inflammation and acidity.

The mental/emotional factors of fear, insecurity, and "holding on" also play a key role in colitis. The mental outlook is directly addressed in reading 278-1 for a 64-year-old librarian. She had had a longstanding condition of chronic mucous colitis accompanied by insomnia, nervousness, and auto-intoxication (a condition in which toxins are reabsorbed, literally poisoning the system as a result of sluggish eliminations. See Chapter 4). She told Cayce she had known for years that there was an imbalance caused by excessive peristalsis in the small intestine and an inactive, crippled colon. She also confessed that she was limited by personal fears and asked how they could be alleviated.

The reading gives several physical remedies, such as Alcaroid for the digestion and hyperacidity, Atomidine to purify the glands, Eno salts for constipation, and low water enemas. However, it was her mental attitude that Cayce considered paramount in her healing. He encouraged her to *know* that everything in her body was being resuscitated back to normal, and to eradicate, in a *positive* manner, any thoughts that interfered with the healing process. He also wrote to her, urging her to hold in her conscious mind the awareness that this was the *right* path, for a positive mental outlook would hasten results.

Again, the most important factor was for her to be persistent and consistent in carrying out the suggestions given.

Later on, she shared that she had fallen into a light sleep during her reading, and was given personal assurance that there is indeed healing in the Divine Presence. She felt that if she could have just held on to that feeling of great hope and inspiration, that the "currents of my physical being would have been radically changed."

She did have difficulty keeping a positive attitude and, within a month, was discouraged by her lack of progress. However, in a second reading, Cayce assured her that progress was, in fact, being made. He again reminded her to have patience and know that her condition could be healed.

Almost two years later, the colitis was not overcome, but had improved. Her spiritual growth had deepened because of her association with Cayce, but she felt she had a long way to go.

What to Do for Colitis

DIET

In a personal letter to Miss 278, following her second reading, Cayce outlined a general diet which had been recommended in several other readings for colitis, digestive upsets, and stomach problems.

Mornings

Citrus fruit or juice (not with cereal)
or
Stewed fruits
or
Dry or cooked cereal (not with citrus)
or
Egg yolks or coddled eggs

Noon

Green salads with any above-ground vegetables that agree with the digestion, such as lettuce, celery, spinach, mustard greens, beans, peas, etc.

Fruit, such as canned peaches, apples, pears, apricots, prunes, etc.

Or the salad may be eaten together with fruit.

Evenings

Cooked vegetables and meats.

In general, Cayce advised limiting sweets, candies, and meat; avoiding pastries; and never eating fried foods. Beef juice was prescribed to strengthen the system. It is easily assimilated and produces a gastric flow through the intestinal tract.

How to Prepare Beef Juice

Note: Chewing the juice before swallowing allows it to be mixed with saliva, stimulating the production of digestive juices.

- Cut 1-1½ pounds round steak (no fat) into ½-inch cubes. Place in a glass canning jar *without* water.
- Place a cloth under the canning jar to prevent breakage, and put the jar in a 2-quart pot.
- Add water so that it comes ¾ of the way up the *outside* of the canning jar and exceeds the level of the beef.
- Cover the jar, but do not seal tightly. Simmer gently for 3-4 hours.
- Strain off the juice, then squeeze any excess juice out of the meat.
- Discard the meat and refrigerate the juice. Do not store for more than 3 days.

To consume

Over a period of 5 minutes, slowly sip 1 tablespoon of beef juice. Repeat this 2-3 times a day. A whole wheat cracker may also be eaten, if desired.

ABDOMINAL GRAPE POULTICE

A poultice is a moist mass of hot or cold herbs or food that is applied to an area of the body for healing.

Occasionally, castor oil packs were prescribed to reduce inflammation, or Epsom salts were suggested to help relax an area of concern, but grape poultices were the most frequently recommended method of treatment for colitis in the readings.

Grapes cleanse and restore the balance in the lymph fluid, dissipate inflammation, and reduce fever.

To make a grape poultice

Crush enough grapes (preferably organic Concord), including skins and seeds, to ultimately cover the abdomen from the ribs to the groin.

Spread a 1-1½ inch layer of crushed grapes between two layers of cheesecloth. Place on the skin, and leave on 4-4½ hours until it becomes as hot as the body. Or make up a fresh poultice every 1–1½ hours until relief is obtained.

Apply daily or weekly, depending on the severity of symptoms.

A TONIC

A 65–year–old female who had chronic colitis (2085) was told that a tonic, taken along with osteopathic adjustments, would gradually correct the colitis. The tonic contains wild ginseng, wild ginger, tincture of stillingia, elixir of lactated pepsin, and grain alcohol.

COLONICS

Colonics are helpful for colitis and may be given with a physician's referral. They are not recommended for ulcerative colitis.

DIARRHEA

Diarrhea is a condition of frequent, watery stools from irritated and inflamed mucous membranes in the intestinal tract. Most simple diarrhea is the result of dietary indiscretions or intestinal flu, and usually lasts 24–48 hours. This is the body's way of quickly ridding itself of an undesirable condition. Diarrhea from food poisoning is far more serious, and a physician should be consulted.

According to Cayce, chronic diarrhea is the result of poor assimilation and an overactive lymph circulation. An incoordination within the nervous system gives the colon mixed messages. As a result, it cannot relax, and frequent, small bowel movements occur that can be distressing and frustrating. The problem is exacerbated by emotional stress, worry, and fear. The fear of losing control happens on other levels, as well, and impatience with the whole problem increases the degree of inflammation.

WHAT TO DO FOR DIARRHEA

1) Castor oil packs for 1–2 hours, 3 to 4 days in a row each week as needed.

2) Colonics, to help remove mucus. Omit the salt/baking soda.

3) Diet:

For Simple Diarrhea: Clear liquids or bulk–forming foods, such as bananas, oatmeal gruel, and rice gruel. Fruits and vegetables can gradually be reintroduced as the stool becomes firm.

For Chronic Diarrhea: Each person must find what foods maintain a proper balance and what foods upset that balance, as underlying causes are gradually corrected.

4) Regular periods of relaxation, visualization, and positive affirmations will bring a calming influence.

Summary

1) Irritable bowel syndrome is a medical term for the syndrome of mucous colitis, spastic colitis, ulcerative colitis, and non-inflammatory diarrhea.

2) Symptoms include diarrhea, constipation, fever, abdominal discomfort, and pain. Bleeding may occur with ulcerative colitis.

3) According to Cayce, colitis is preceded by a cold or intestinal flu that disturbs the intestinal lymphatics.

4) Fear, insecurity, and difficulty in "letting go" are underlying issues to consider.

5) Follow a moderate diet. Beef juice is recommended as a medicinal food to stimulate the gastric flow and strengthen the system.

6) Abdominal grape poultices cleanse the lymph, reduce fever, and heal inflammation.

7) Simple diarrhea usually lasts 24–48 hours.

8) Chronic diarrhea stems from an overactive lymph, poor assimilation, and negative emotions.

9) Castor oil packs, colonics, diet guidelines, relaxation, and visualization all help in correcting the situation.

TWELVE

Parasites and Candida

Hence we would continue the care as to activities related to the diet, as related to associations with others, as related to the abuses of influences in filling the system with destructive forces; and we will find we will keep for this body a continuity not only of the re-creative force within self, but of the vital active forces in same.

1554-4

Parasites

A parasite is an organism that lives within or upon another organism and receives its nourishment at the expense of the host. Some parasites excrete harmful toxins, and others cause injury to the intestinal wall. Over 20 million Americans are infected with some form of worm or parasite.

Parasites are transmitted through contaminated food and drinking water, infected soil, and infected stools of man and animals (the transmission from animals is most often from domestic pets). Although parasites can be present in the intestinal tract without showing up in fecal matter, a diagnosis can usually be made from three fresh stool specimens. These should, ideally, be examined within 30 minutes of being collected.

Dr. Jensen, an iridologist introduced in Chapter 4, agrees that worms are commonly found in the intestinal tract, and attributes the type of parasite to the amount and type of toxic material present. Some people who have parasites and/or worms will have no symptoms, while others will complain of diarrhea, fever, cramping, anal itching, bloody stools, nausea/vomiting, and an inabililty to digest food.

There are several methods of treatment, including pharmaceutical drugs, homeopathic remedies, and herbs such as raw garlic, pumpkin seeds, and black walnut tincture. Having a colonic once a week or enemas twice a week is recommended during a treatment program to flush out the parasites.

PREVENTION

- A good, thorough, daily elimination is very important. Parasites thrive when the passage of stool slows down, allowing time for their eggs to hatch.
- Wash hands before handling and preparing food.
- Carefully and thoroughly wash all raw food to eliminate any parasite eggs.
- Eat plentiful amounts of raw garlic (parasites dislike the odor), raw cabbage, and leafy green vegetables.
- Avoid mucus–forming food, such as wheat and dairy, for parasites burrow into the built–up mucous lining of the intestinal tract.
- Maintain a healthy, alkaline 7.4 pH of the blood by eating an 80% alkaline/20% acid diet, for acidity invites parasites.
- Avoid raw fish/sushi.
- Thoroughly cook all fish, poultry, lamb, beef, and pork (although Cayce did not advocate eating pork, except for crisp bacon).
- Drink distilled, bottled water when traveling or camping, and avoid ice cubes because they may be made from contaminated water.
- Be aware of any attitude that allows us to leave ourselves open to outside influences that may invade, inhibit, or devitalize our mental and physical health.

CLASSIFICATIONS

There are five major classifications of parasites: Protozoa, Flatworms, Roundworms, Thorny-headed worms, and Anthropoda, the latter two being rather uncommon. We will discuss seven of the most common varieties.

Protozoa: amoeba, giardia

Flatworm: dwarf tapeworm

Roundworm: common roundworm, pinworm, whipworm, hook-worm

PROTOZOA: Amoeba

Entamoeba histolytica are one-celled organisms, averaging 20 microns in diameter, that live primarily in the large intestine. They penetrate the

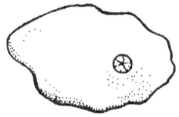

mucous lining, form ulcers, and feed on red blood cells. They may or may not cause discomfort; however, amoebic dysentery causes pain, cramping, gas, bloody stools, mucus, loss of appetite, weight loss, and chronic fatigue. Entamoeba histolytica are more common in rural areas, countries with poor sanitation, and where there are crowded living conditions, such as prisons and asylums.

PROTOZOA: Giardia

Giardia lamblia are intestinal flagellates, 9–21 microns long, that are found in the upper part of the small intestine and gallbladder. They move erratically, and can lodge throughout the system, making them difficult to treat. They cause a widespread variety of symptoms, including mild diarrhea, gas, lack of appetite, crampy abdominal pain, and general toxicity. They are becoming a serious public health problem, for many cities have drinking water that is contaminated with giardia.

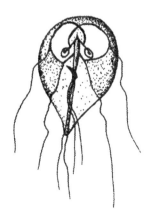

FLATWORM (Cestodes)

There are many flat and segmented varieties of flatworm, measuring up to several meters in length. One can get tapeworms (one kind of flatworm) by eating raw or undercooked fish, pork, or beef. If the eggs 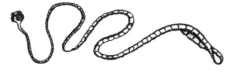 are swallowed, they hatch in the small intestine, attach to the villi with suckers, and absorb food. With a heavy infestation, one may experience diarrhea, abdominal pain, headache, dizziness, weight loss, or a lack of appetite.

A 37-year-old woman (602) asked Cayce if there were any indication of tapeworms in her body. She was told "not as yet," but that the conditions for this to happen exist in every person. He went on to explain that one body lives upon another in every form of existence, and the human body has its parasites both internally and externally.

A 26-year-old man (567-7) was told that he could test himself for tapeworms by going on a three-day apple diet, followed by a half teacup of olive oil. If he indeed had tapeworms, they would be present and visible in his stool after the three-day period.

Dr. Bernard Jensen, in *The Science and Practice of Iridology*, gives the following directions for eliminating tapeworms:

> The patient must eat nothing but garlic or onions for two days. Then a powerful herbal laxative is given, and when it is time for the bowel to evacuate, the patient sits in a vessel of warm milk. Since cold air usually keeps the worm from leaving the body, the warm milk is a favorable means of getting it to pass out of the lower bowel. (p. 358)

ROUNDWORM (Nematodes)

There are over 500,000 species of roundworms in the world, but only four will be considered here. The female is much larger than the male, and can average 20-35 centimeters in length. They are usually a light, creamy-white color, although the female may appear darker when filled with eggs.

COMMON ROUNDWORM

Ascaris lumbricoides, or common roundworm, lives in the small intestine, but the eggs migrate to the liver, heart, and lungs when first ingested. 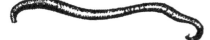 They are contracted from poor sanitation, infected food or drink, or by inhalation. People who have roundworms are often asymptomatic; however, when large numbers of roundworms are present, there may be an allergic reaction.

PINWORM

The pinworm, *enterobius vermicularis*, is 8–13 millimeters long, and commonly found in children throughout the world. Pinworms do not attach to the lining of the intestine; the female migrates to the anus at night, where she deposits her eggs. The newborn worms cause anal itching, which is often the most uncomfortable symptom. Pinworms are easily transmitted through bed linens, clothing, toys, infected soil, and infected stool.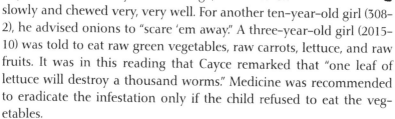

Cayce gave 28 readings on this subject. For a ten-year-old girl (1401-2), he advised that for one whole day, she receive only raw cabbage, to be eaten slowly and chewed very, very well. For another ten-year-old girl (308-2), he advised onions to "scare 'em away." A three-year-old girl (2015-10) was told to eat raw green vegetables, raw carrots, lettuce, and raw fruits. It was in this reading that Cayce remarked that "one leaf of lettuce will destroy a thousand worms." Medicine was recommended to eradicate the infestation only if the child refused to eat the vegetables.

A five-year-old boy (2542-4) was so infested that he gritted his teeth in his sleep (a common symptom), caught colds easily, and had a rash all over his face and body. The overwhelming number of pinworms had thinned the intestinal wall, allowing toxins to seep into the blood and be eliminated through the skin rather than the colon. The toxins were so irritating that they caused a skin rash. The boy was advised not to have sweets until the worms were eradicated.

Although we generally think of pinworms as a problem predominantly in children, Cayce says there is matter in *everyone's* intestinal tract that produces a form of worm when milk containing bacillus is consumed.

Reading 1597-2 is an unusual case of a 32-year-old man who suffered from dizziness, hot and cold flushes, phlegm in the throat, coughing spells at bedtime, and eye pain. He told Cayce that he had eaten dirt as a youngster, and wanted to know if that had any bearing on his present health problems. The reading does not directly address his concern over this, but it seems highly likely that it was a factor in his parasitic condition. In his physical evaluation, Cayce found that a form of pinworm was indeed responsible for the man's numerous and valid complaints. The pinworms even attacked his liver and kidneys at times and affected the eliminations. He was told to go on an apple diet for three days, and take one-half teacup of pure olive oil on the third evening to remove the cause of the disturbance.

WHIPWORM

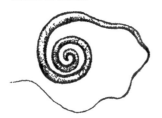

The eggs of the whipworm, *trichuris trichiura*, find their way into the colon, especially the cecum and appendix. The mature worm attaches to the intestinal wall, where it causes inflammation and, occasionally, appendicitis. The female is about 3-5 centimeters long.

HOOKWORM

Both the Old World hookworm, *Ancylostoma duodenale*, and the New World hookworm, *Necator americanus*, are grayish-white or pink, and one centimeter long. Their eggs grow and develop in soil, and pen-

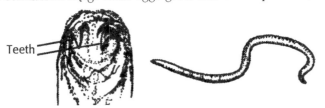

Teeth

etrate one's feet when walking barefoot in infected soil. Hookworms have teeth that attach to the wall of the intestines, and cause lesions as they suck the blood and tissue.

Candida

Many people who have parasites and worms also frequently have a problem with systemic Candida. *Candida albicans* are fungal micro-flora found almost everywhere. For example, they are paramount in the fermentation and aging process of beer, wine, yogurt, cheese, vinegar, bread, and other foods, and co-exist with friendly lactobacilli in the mouth, throat, and colon. When an overgrowth of Candida occurs in a person, the fungus can leave the intestinal tract and become systemic by spreading, via the blood, to the liver, heart, lungs, and other organs. In recent years, systemic Candida has grown into a serious health problem because of many factors: more stressful lifestyles that affect the immune system, poor nutrition, overuse of antibiotics, etc. There are no readings on the subject because it was not a health concern at that time.

There are two tests for Candida, though they are not completely reliable: a blood test for the presence of certain antibodies, and a stool exam to determine the presence of Candida in the intestinal tract.

CANDIDA SYMPTOMS
- Abdominal bloating, heartburn, and indigestion
- Craving for sweets
- Poor attention span; memory loss
- Mood swings, depression, anxiety, fatigue
- Constipation, diarrhea, bad breath
- Dizziness, headaches
- Bladder infections
- PMS symptoms, increased craving for sweets before menstruation, vaginal yeast discharge

CAUSES OF CANDIDA
1) *Antibiotics* destroy not only the harmful bacteria in the body, but the beneficial bacteria as well. Acidophilus is one such helpful bacteria that keeps Candida in check. One should be cautious about the consumption of poultry, pigs, and cows, for they are routinely given antibiotics.
2) *Birth control pills.*

3) *Drugs.* Cortisone, in particular, suppresses the immune system and contributes to the overgrowth of Candida.

4) *Prolonged exposure to environmental hazards.* Mold, mildew, chemicals, pollutants, noise stress, and pesticides all lower the effectiveness of the immune system.

5) *Negative attitudes and emotions.* Candida overgrowth is facilitated by worry, obsession over the past, perfectionism, feeling scattered, and by repressed emotions.

6) *Direct infection* from catheterizations, dialysis, intravenous feedings, and surgery.

7) *Diet.* Candida feeds on sugar, sweeteners, wheat, and processed foods. A healthy intestinal tract needs fermented food to support and maintain friendly bacteria. When being treated for Candida, however, all potentially fermentation–producing foods should be avoided.

Fermentation-Producing Foods

    Bread
    Alcoholic beverages
    Aged cheese
    Yogurt, kefir, sour cream, buttermilk
    Pickles, mustard, catsup, relish, vinegar
    Miso, soy sauce
    Tofu, tempeh
    Sauerkraut (raw is okay)
    Mushrooms
    Cider
    Processed meats (sausage, bacon, cold cuts, ham, hot dogs, etc.)

TREATMENT FOR CANDIDA

1) Destroy the overgrowth of yeast with pharmaceutical drugs or homeopathic remedies or herbs such as Pau d'Arco and garlic.

2) Restore the balance of the intestinal flora by taking acidophilus liquid or capsules (not yogurt, kefir, or Rejuvelac, which are fermented foods).

3) During a treatment program, have colonics to clean out the toxins from dead yeast cells. Die–off symptoms, such as nausea, depression, headaches, skin rash, foggy thinking, poor memory, muscle and

joint pain, or flu-like symptoms occur most often during the second to fifth day of treatment and last for one to two weeks.

4)   Boost the immune system with castor oil packs and herbs such as echinacea, astragalus, and Pau d'Arco.

5)   Diet. Eliminate the following foods/drinks for one month:

- Salads and other raw, cold food
- Breads, cookies, cakes, pasta
- Fermentation-producing food (see list on page 144)
- Beef, pork, chicken
- Fruit (except tropical fruit)
- Dairy products
- Peanuts, pistachios
- Leftovers
- Coffee, tea (except Pau d'Arco)
- Sodas
- Alcoholic beverages
- Sugar and sweeteners

What To Eat/Drink For One Month:

- 6–8 glasses of water daily
- Pau d'Arco or black walnut tea
- Corn, rice, buckwheat, quinoa, millet, amaranth
- Beans and legumes
- Vegetables (Limit lima beans, white potatoes, winter squash, lentils, pumpkin, and peas.)
- Seafood
- Raw, unsalted nuts (except peanuts and pistachios)
- Seeds (sunflower, sesame, pumpkin)
- Raw sauerkraut (not canned or pasteurized)
- Eggs and unsalted butter
- Brewer's yeast (This is a species different from other yeasts, and does not cause a problem unless there is a general allergy to *all* yeasts.)
- Tropical fruits (pineapple, papaya, mango, kiwi, bananas) if eaten once a day and not combined with other food.

(There is some disagreement over the use of tropical fruits. A few authorities advise eliminating all fruit, because mold grows on the fruit's skin. Cantaloupes, berries, and grapes mold quickly and should be freshly picked. And since sugar is a primary food for yeast, there is also some concern over the sugar content of fruit.)

After one month on a Candida elimination diet, gradually reintroduce one food per week that has been omitted. Sugar, beer, wine, liquor, and dairy should be introduced last. Watch for such adverse reactions as headache, bloating, or sudden fatigue. Each person will need to individualize the diet for maximum health. Yeast is always present in the body, but will no longer cause problems once the system is rebalanced.

The following books are recommended for further study:

Candida, by Luc De Schepper, M.D., which was the primary source for this chapter.

The Yeast Syndrome, by John Parks Trowbridge, M.D., and Morton Walker, D.P.M.

The Yeast Connection, by William G. Crook, M.D.

Summary

1) Parasites are transmitted via contaminated food and drinking water, infected soil, and the infected stools of man and animals.

2) Standard treatment is either pharmaceutical medicine or homeopathic remedies or herbs.

3) An infestation of parasites can be prevented by having thorough, daily eliminations; proper hand-washing; thoroughly cooking beef, pork, and fish; washing raw food before eating; drinking distilled, bottled water when traveling; avoiding ice cubes; and by transforming one's negative attitudes.

4) The presence of parasites may be asymptomatic or may cause diarrhea, fever, loss of appetite, nausea/vomiting, bloody stools, cramping, and may prevent food from being properly digested.

5) Systemic Candida has become a serious threat to our health.

6) The major causes of Candida are the use of antibiotics, birth control pills, drugs that suppress the immune system, negative attitudes, prolonged exposure to environmental hazards, and a diet high in sugar, wheat, and fermented or processed foods.

7) Symptoms vary, but will generally include abdominal bloating, heartburn, indigestion, craving for sweets, poor attention span, memory loss, and mood swings.

8) Treatment consists of destroying the overgrowth of Candida, restoring the acidophilus balance, having a series of colonics, boosting the immune system, and following a yeast-free diet for one month. Body-building foods that were originally omitted from the diet because of their yeast-encouraging qualities may then be gradually reintroduced.

Closing Thoughts

Cayce truly understood that the foundation for health, vitality, and even longevity is a clean colon and thorough daily eliminations.

It requires ongoing attention to stay healthy, for it is really a state of balance that is *our* responsibility. We decide how much sleep to get, when to exercise, what foods should be eaten, what our lifestyle will be, etc. Everything we do affects us and ultimately reaches the colon. It needs regular care and nurturing, just like any other part of the body. As Cayce put it so well:

> And the keeping of the colon clean is that which is necessary for *every* well-balanced body.   1703-2

APPENDIX

Excerpts from Two Readings

EXCERPT FROM READING 457-11
(Female, age 34)

25. (Q) Has blood pressure really gone down so much?
(A) It is very little above normal at present.

26. (Q) What caused it to go down? The vacation with its unusual amount of exercise and fresh air?
(A) The cleansing of the body forces. This, from this body, is produced from a colon irritation.

28. (Q) Are there any specific suggestions for osteopathic treatments now?
(A) The relaxing of the muscular forces, not stimulating but relaxing of the muscular forces from the lumbar axis to the 6th and 7th dorsal.

29. (Q) What causes the gray film on teeth?
(A) The chemical balance in the system and the throw–off or discharge from breath in the lungs. This is a source from which drosses are relieved from the system, and thus passing through the teeth produce same on the teeth. Keeping such cleansed with an equal combination of soda and salt at least three to four times a week will cleanse these of

this disturbance. The use of Ipsab as a wash for mouth and gums will further aid in keeping these conditions cleansed; and any good dentifrice once or twice a day.

EXCERPT FROM READING 191-1
(Female, age 25)

1. EC: We have the body here, [191]. Now, we find there are specific disorders accentuated in the physical forces of this body, and these may be corrected in such a manner as to bring a normal physical functioning. The conditions, as we find, have to do with eliminations, the effect same has produced on specific organs and the result of this effect.

2. These, then, are the conditions as we find them with this body, [191] we are speaking of, present in this room.

3. First, in the *blood supply*—here we find the conditions are an over-taxed blood supply, through the manner in which eliminations have been carried on in the system. This leaving drosses, especially in the alimentary canal, affecting directly the liver, and this re-infection, as it were, from the poisons in system, produces an over-abundance of the blood supply so contaminated, as it were, in the throat, the bronchia, the larynx, the pounding to the head, and the flow becomes such as to produce temperature in the blood supply. This from the character of the dross accumulation, produces in the blood stream and not sufficient of the leucocyte that destroys the tissue that becomes involved—and is carried off, or *should* be carried off, in elimination.

4. In the *nerve system*—this, we find, becomes taxed through the over supply of blood from the solar plexus *upward*, especially—and at times causes both sympathetically and specifically, ganglia to work in an extraordinary, or an abnormal manner. Hence the fast pulsations as felt in the upper portion of body, through head, through neck, at times even in the palms of hand; yet the tendency in the lower portion to feel chilly, with hot and cold sensation. These are reflexes from sympathetic and nerve plexus in the cerebrospinal system.

5. In the functionings of the *organs*, these show specific conditions as exist—in that of the pressure in head, causing headaches, that take peculiar *turns*, as it were, through the head. Eyes at times burn, *without*

any *particular* effect to vision. Throat irritation. Larynx—this shows the greater effect of the plethora condition existent in the upper portion of system, or the radiation of the blood supply above the diaphragm. Inflammation ensues from same. Lungs themselves very good, though soreness naturally occurs from the feeling of irritation in the bronchia and larynx. In the digestive system, with the blood supply above the diaphragm—naturally the digestion becomes poor, and insufficient activity carried on. The condition in *liver*, sluggish in its activity—with the tendency towards the *inactivity* of the bile ducts, as also of the spleen's reflexes in the activity of digestion. Hepatic circulation becomes cold, or slow so that the tendency is the *over* crowding of the lower hepatic circulation, and the inactivity of same.

6. To meet the needs of the conditions, so that there *is* the *permanent* elimination of the disorders from the system:

First we would use those of an *eliminant* that will cause activity within the blood stream proper, and the causing of an activity in the hepatic circulation as to produce a normal return of the plasm in the division of the blood supply, producing an activity in the liver at the same time. These we would find in this, and we would take three of these, one day apart; that is, take one—rest a day and then take the next—rest a day, taking the next—see?

> Podophyllin.............. ½ grain,
> Leptandrin .... ¼ grain,
> Sanguinaria .... ¼ grain.

This should be put in capsule, and this divided into the three doses, see? To add with this, as the *carrier*, we would take those of the Cascara Sagrada ½ grain, making then the capsule of the whole amount into three divisions, after they are well compounded.

7. Following this, we would use—or use throughout—those of the inhalant as would be prepared in *this* manner: To 4 ounces of grain alcohol, in an 8 ounce container, add:

> Oil of Eucalyptol...20 minims,
> Rectified Creosote ....5 minims,
> Benzoin ....5 minims,
> Rectified Oil of Turp ....5 minims,
> Tincture of Tolu in solution ....30 minims.

Shake solution together when it is to be inhaled. Keep this in a glass corked container. Inhale *through* the mouth, principally, into the lungs and larynx. This may be taken often when coughing, or when irritation of the throat or of the larynx occurs, and will *prevent* coughing. Do not inhale too deep in the beginning. Will also be well that this be inhaled (shaken each time before it is inhaled) through the nostrils. This will clarify the condition in the head and reduce the pressure to the soft tissue of face and head.

8.   Well that each evening, before retiring, the feet—to the knees—be bathed in hot water, to which *mustard* is added.

To the gallon of water, half a teaspoonful of mustard—rubbing in the sole of the feet, following same, those of mutton tallow and camphorated oil. This acts in *this* manner: This will produce a circulation through the extremities that, added with the stimuli to the hepatic circulation, will aid in *equalizing* and caring for the conditions as *produce* drosses in the body.

Resources

Edgar Cayce's A.R.E.
Association for Research and Enlightenment
(800) 333-4499
EdgarCayce.org

•

A.R.E. Health Center and Spa
(757) 457-7202
email: Spa@EdgarCayce.org

•

The Cayce/Reilly® School of Massage
(757) 457-7270
email: info @caycereilly.edu

•

All located at:
215 67th Street, Virginia Beach, VA 23451–2061

Also click on *Holistic Health* at EdgarCayce.org

References

Bieler, Henry G., M.D. *Food Is Your Best Medicine.* New York: Random House, Inc., 1968.

Bolton, Brett, ed. *Edgar Cayce Speaks.* New York: Avon Books, 1969.

De Schepper, Luc, M.D., Ph.D, C.A. *Candida.* Santa Monica, CA: Dr. Luc DeSchepper, 1986.

Edgar Cayce Foundation. *An Edgar Cayce Home Medicine Guide.* Virginia Beach, VA: A.R.E. Press, 1982.

Goodman, Saul. *The Book of Shiatzu.* Garden City Park, NY: Avery Publishing Group, 1990.

Gray, Robert. *The Colon Health Handbook.* Reno, NV: Emerald Publishing, 1986.

Jensen, Bernard, D.C., N.D. *Foods that Heal.* Garden City Park, NY: Avery Publishing Group, 1988.

——. *The Science and Practice of Iridology.* Escondido, CA: Jensen's Nutritional and Health Products, 1952.

——. with Sylvia Bell. *Tissue Cleansing through Bowel Management.* Escondido, CA: Bernard Jensen, 1981.

McGarey, William A., M.D. *The Oil that Heals.* Virginia Beach, VA: A.R.E. Press, 1993.

Markell, Edward, Ph.D, M.D., and Marietta Voge, MA, Ph.D. *Medical Parasitology.* Philadelphia: W.B. Saunders Co., 1976.

Mein, Eric, M.D. *Keys to Health: The Promise and Challenge of Holism.* New York: Harper & Row, 1989.

Pagano, John, D.C. *Healing Psoriasis.* Englewood Cliffs, NJ: The Pagano Organization, 1991.

Reilly, Harold J., D.Ph.T., D.S., and Ruth Hagy Brod. *The Edgar Cayce Handbook for Health through Drugless Therapy.* Virginia Beach, VA: A.R.E. Press, 1975.

Tilden, J.H., M.D. *Toxemia Explained.* New Canaan, CT: Keats Publishing, Inc., 1976.

Walker, Norman, D.Sc., Ph.D. *Colon Health.* Phoenix, AZ: O'Sullivan Woodside & Co., 1979.

Wright, Machaelle Small. *Flower Essences.* Jeffersonton, VA: Perelandra, Ltd, 1988.

Index

A

B

99, 111, 143–144
Bactericide 63
Bad breath 33, 143
Baking soda 84, 86, 92–93, 96, 101, 133
Ballooning (of the colon) 103
Bananas 51, 53, 112, 122, 134, 145
Beans 48–49, 56, 112, 122, 131, 145
Beef 48, 132, 138, 140, 145, 147
Beef juice 31, 109, 131–132, 135
Beer 143, 146
Beets 13, 15, 49
Below–ground vegetables 45, 48–49
Bentonite 40
Bieler, Henry M.D. 35, 79, 157
Bifidus, L. 14
Bile 13, 23, 33, 36, 104, 107, 117, 125, 153
Birth control pills 143, 147
Black walnut tea 145
Black walnut tincture 138
Bladder 114, 143
Bleach bath (for fruits and vegetables) 62
Bleeding 91, 110, 123, 135
Bloating 100, 143, 146–147
Blood 13, 16–17, 23, 33–36, 39–41, 44, 46, 48, 55, 58, 61, 63, 72, 79, 83, 89, 101, 106, 126, 138–139, 141–142, 147, 152–153
Blood–building (foods) 44, 55
Blood circulation 16–17, 20, 24, 34, 49, 62, 72, 74–75, 77, 90, 116, 120, 153, 154
Blood circulaton and massage 62
Blood pH 55–58, 79, 138
Blood pressure 37, 48, 61, 71–72, 74, 81, 93, 116, 151
Blood purifiers 46, 89, 101
Blood test (Candida) 143
Blood vessels 17, 61
Bloody stools 138–139
Boils 35, 126
Bowel 87, 126
Bowel movement 12, 14, 99, 107, 110, 119, 133
Brandt, Joanna 63
Breach–beating 76–77, 81

Bread 48, 50, 53–54, 111, 143–145
Breakfast 16, 44, 57, 124
Breast milk 37
Breath, shortness of 12, 16, 75, 108
Breathing 17, 21, 62, 71, 96, 101, 154
Breathing, deep 17, 21, 62, 96, 101, 154
Brevis, L. 14
Brewer's yeast 145
Broccoli 49, 112
Bronchitis 35
Broth 53, 109
Bulgaris, L. 14
Bulk–forming (laxatives) 122–123
Bursitis 2–4, 9, 90
Butter 44, 145
Buttocks 77

C

Cabbage 49, 53, 112, 138, 141
Caffeine (*See also coffee, tea*) 12, 64
Cancer 12, 30, 39, 45, 63, 91, 116, 121
Candida 14, 40, 137, 143–144, 146, 147, 157
Canker sores 31
Cantaloupe 51, 146
Carbolic acid 110
Carbon (ash) 34
Carbon dioxide 34
Carbonated drinks 16, 54
Cardiac disease (*See also heart*) 91
Carob 122
Caroid Laxative 125
Caroid and Bile Salts 125
Carrot juice 107, 120–121, 127
Carrots 44, 46, 49, 51, 141
Cascara Sagrada 125, 153
Castor oil 3, 24, 85, 87, 93–95, 100–101, 107, 109, 111–113, 117, 120, 123–124, 132–133, 135, 145
Castor oil packs 3, 24, 93, 100–101, 107, 109, 111, 113–114, 117, 132–133, 135, 145
Catarrh 36
Cathartics 119–120, 127
Catheterizations 144
Cauliflower 49, 112

121, 125, 130–131, 153
Digestive enzymes 14, 16, 23, 50
Dinner 45
Disease 11, 21, 35, 37, 39, 40, 75, 90, 103
Disposable hoses 89
Diverticula 113, 117
Diverticulitis 17, 21, 103, 113–114, 117
Diverticulosis 91, 103, 113, 114, 117
Dizziness 36, 75, 116, 140, 142–143
Dorsals 74
Double-knee kiss (exercise) 18
Drafts 79
Dreams 41, 42
Drosses (*See also toxins*) 33, 35, 151–152, 154
Drugs (prescription) 7, 34, 56, 100, 138, 144, 147
Duodenum 23, 109, 125

E

E. coli 14
Ears 4, 9
Ebers Papyrus 32
Echinacea 145
Eczema 108, 126
Eggs
    Egg whites 45, 56
    Egg yolks 44–45, 56, 131
Eggs (parasite) 138, 140–142
Egypt, Egyptian 1, 32, 121
Elbow-knee kiss (exercise) 18
Electrolytes 25
Eliminant (=laxative) 119–120, 122, 153
Eliminations 2, 8, 9, 11–13, 16–17, 23, 26, 32–35, 37, 42, 46, 49, 56, 58, 72, 76–77, 80, 84, 90, 103, 106, 121–122, 126, 130, 142, 147, 149, 152
Elixir of lactated pepsin 133
Elliot machine 78
Emotions 3, 9, 50, 56, 76, 78–79, 104, 106, 108, 112, 117, 135, 144
Enema effect 90
Enemas 12, 21, 30, 38, 61, 77, 84, 92,

130, 138
Enemas, other types
    Coffee 85, 101
    Colema 87, 101
    High enema (colon tube) 86, 101
    Medicated 86, 101
    Oil retention 86, 101
    Three-stage 86, 101
Energy 4, 7, 9, 17, 41, 50–51, 52, 62, 90, 97, 106, 107
Engorgement (of the colon) 8, 75, 77, 81
Eno Salts 12, 14, 16, 23, 50, 126, 130
Epsom Salts 61, 77, 120, 132
Esophagus 23
Essenes 32, 42
Esssential oils 62
Exercise(s) 2, 12, 17, 20–21, 30, 55, 60, 62, 71, 89, 99, 100, 104, 106–107, 115, 117, 122, 149, 151
Eyes 35, 37, 40, 46, 60, 90, 100, 142, 152

F

Fasting, (Chapter 6) 34, 40–42, 59–64, 68, 84, 86, 90
Fatigue 56, 62, 99, 139, 143, 146
Fats 24, 33, 77–78
Fear 8, 45, 79, 108, 114, 130, 133, 135
Fecal 4, 13, 63, 86, 91, 113, 117, 137
Feet 4, 9, 77, 79, 110, 115–116, 126, 142, 154
Fermentation, fermented foods 14, 92, 109, 111, 121, 143–145, 147
Fever 13, 21, 35, 113, 117, 129, 132, 135, 138, 147
Fiber 11, 30, 58, 104, 107, 113, 117
Figs 120–121, 127
Filtration (by the liver) 33, 35
Fish 17, 31, 45, 48, 53, 56, 99, 109, 138, 140, 147
Fistula (anal) 91
Flatulence (*See also gas*) 111, 117
Flatworms 139–140
Fletcher's Castoria 124
Flour 12, 53, 56, 93, 99, 114, 122

Y

Yeast 14, 40, 144–147
Yellow–colored foods 51
Yoga abdominal lift 107, 115
Yogurt 14, 99, 143, 144

Z

Zilatone 125

A.R.E. PRESS

Edgar Cayce (1877–1945) founded the non-profit Association for Research and Enlightenment (A.R.E.) in 1931, to explore spirituality, holistic health, intuition, dream interpretation, psychic development, reincarnation, and ancient mysteries—all subjects that frequently came up in the more than 14,000 documented psychic readings given by Cayce.

Edgar Cayce's A.R.E. provides individuals from all walks of life and a variety of religious backgrounds with tools for personal transformation and healing at all levels—body, mind, and spirit.

A.R.E. Press has been publishing since 1931 as well, with the mission of furthering the work of A.R.E. by publishing books, DVDs, and CDs to support the organization's goal of helping people to change their lives for the better physically, mentally, and spiritually.

In 2009, A.R.E. Press launched its second imprint, 4th Dimension Press. While A.R.E. Press features topics directly related to the work of Edgar Cayce and often includes excerpts from the Cayce readings, 4th Dimension Press allows us to take our publishing efforts further with like-minded and expansive explorations into the mysteries and spirituality of our existence without direct reference to Cayce-specific content.

**A.R.E. Press/4th Dimension Press
215 67th Street
Virginia Beach, VA 23451**

Learn more at EdgarCayce.org. Visit ARECatalog.com to browse and purchase additional titles.

ARE PRESS.COM

BAAR PRODUCTS

A.R.E.'s Official Worldwide Exclusive Supplier of Edgar Cayce Health Care Products

Baar Products, Inc., is the official worldwide exclusive supplier of Edgar Cayce health care products. Baar offers a collection of natural products and remedies drawn from the work of Edgar Cayce, considered by many to be the father of modern holistic medicine.

For a complete listing of Cayce-related products, call:

800-269-2502

Or write:

**Baar Products, Inc.
P.O. Box 60
Downingtown, PA 19335 U.S.A.
Customer Service and International: 610-873-4591
Fax: 610-873-7945
Web Site: www.baar.com   E-mail: cayce@baar.com**

EDGAR CAYCE'S A.R.E.

Who Was Edgar Cayce?
Twentieth Century Psychic and Medical Clairvoyant

Edgar Cayce (pronounced Kay-Cee, 1877-1945) has been called the "sleeping prophet," the "father of holistic medicine," and the most-documented psychic of the 20th century. For more than 40 years of his adult life, Cayce gave psychic "readings" to thousands of seekers while in an unconscious state, diagnosing illnesses and revealing lives lived in the past and prophecies yet to come. But who, exactly, was Edgar Cayce?

Cayce was born on a farm in Hopkinsville, Kentucky, in 1877, and his psychic abilities began to appear as early as his childhood. He was able to see and talk to his late grandfather's spirit, and often played with "imaginary friends" whom he said were spirits on the other side. He also displayed an uncanny ability to memorize the pages of a book simply by sleeping on it. These gifts labeled the young Cayce as strange, but all Cayce really wanted was to help others, especially children.

Later in life, Cayce would find that he had the ability to put himself into a sleep-like state by lying down on a couch, closing his eyes, and folding his hands over his stomach. In this state of relaxation and meditation, he was able to place his mind in contact with all time and space—the universal consciousness, also known as the super-conscious mind. From there, he could respond to questions as broad as, "What are the secrets of the universe?" and "What is my purpose in life?" to as specific as, "What can I do to help my arthritis?" and "How were the pyramids of Egypt built?" His responses to these questions came to be called "readings," and their insights offer practical help and advice to individuals even today.

The majority of Edgar Cayce's readings deal with holistic health and the treatment of illness. Yet, although best known for this material, the sleeping Cayce did not seem to be limited to concerns about the physical body. In fact, in their entirety, the readings discuss an astonishing 10,000 different topics. This vast array of subject matter can be narrowed down into a smaller group of topics that, when compiled together, deal with the following five categories: (1) Health-Related Information; (2) Philosophy and Reincarnation; (3) Dreams and Dream Interpretation; (4) ESP and Psychic Phenomena; and (5) Spiritual Growth, Meditation, and Prayer.

Learn more at EdgarCayce.org.

What Is A.R.E.?

Edgar Cayce founded the non-profit Association for Research and Enlightenment (A.R.E.) in 1931, to explore spirituality, holistic health, intuition, dream interpretation, psychic development, reincarnation, and ancient mysteries—all subjects that frequently came up in the more than 14,000 documented psychic readings given by Cayce.

The Mission of the A.R.E. is to help people transform their lives for the better, through research, education, and application of core concepts found in the Edgar Cayce readings and kindred materials that seek to manifest the love of God and all people and promote the purposefulness of life, the oneness of God, the spiritual nature of humankind, and the connection of body, mind, and spirit.

With an international headquarters in Virginia Beach, Va., a regional headquarters in Houston, regional representatives throughout the U.S., Edgar Cayce Centers in more than thirty countries, and individual members in more than seventy countries, the A.R.E. community is a global network of individuals.

A.R.E. conferences, international tours, camps for children and adults, regional activities, and study groups allow like-minded people to gather for educational and fellowship opportunities worldwide.

A.R.E. offers membership benefits and services that include a quarterly body-mind-spirit member magazine, *Venture Inward*, a member newsletter covering the major topics of the readings, and access to the entire set of readings in an exclusive online database.

Learn more at EdgarCayce.org.

EDGARCAYCE.ORG